When
Sleeping Beauty
Wakes Up

When
Sleeping Beauty
Wakes Up

A Woman's Tale
of Healing the Immune System
and Awakening the Feminine

Patt Lind-Kyle

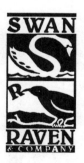

Swan • Raven and Company
1427 NW 23rd Avenue, Suite 8
Portland, Oregon 97210
(800) 488-4849

Published by Swan • Raven & Company,
1427 NW 23rd Avenue, Suite 8, Portland, Oregon 97210
(800) 488-4849

Library of Congress # 92-93335 Catalog Card Number:
ISBN 0-9632310-1-4 $14.95 Ordering information in
rear of book.

Cover design and illustration by Marcia Barrentine

Book design by The Write Touch, Sally R. Petersen

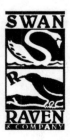

CONTENTS

ACKNOWLEDGMENTS

I want to acknowledge CFIDS for stopping the normal flow of my life and taking me on an incredible awakening journey. I would like to thank some of the healers who joined me long the way; Murina Bokelman, John Mayfield D.C. , Steven Banaster, M.D., Gary Gordon M.D., Stephen Barr, L.Ac., Patty Keeney, Corrie Upham, Georgia Dow, Marilyn Nyborg, Sharyn McDonald, Gail and Marilyn Youngbird. My biggest applause is to my husband David Kyle without whose constant loyalty, inspiration and love, I would not have returned from this journey with such sacred treasures. And to our daughter Shellie Sever for her loving presence that led to my vision.

In birthing this book I could not have done it without my editor Myrna Oakley who worked long and hard under a tight time schedule. I am thankful to Chrystal Harves, Elaine Walsh, and Ruby Allen who shared their clarity and insightful suggestions and Scott Taylor for illustration ideas. Marcia Barrentine for her magnificent cover, the creative visual image of today's Professional Awakened Sleeping Beauty. To David for his editing and encouragement. And, finally, Sally Petersen, who masterfully orchestrated this book into print.

A special thank you to each woman in the research project, who gave her time, openly shared her life stories, and her wisdom, from which I gained a knowledge of the feminine, and a connection to myself.

FOREWORD

The reader is about to embark upon a profound journey. Traveling by rollercoaster, you will descend into a kind of quiet hell, to re-emerge only after having tasted not just the pain of the author's struggle with an illness, but also, her search for self-knowledge, autonomy, meaning, and personal empowerment.

As a woman's advocate, it has been my life's work to ensure that women have access to power and independence — economic equality, political power, educational opportunity, and cultural respect. Nevertheless, the complex integration of social oppression and physical health is a topic that has rarely been explored in such a thorough and intimate way as Patt Lind-Kyle does with this book. Hers is not only a literal story of her battle with a "woman's disease," but also a metaphorical telling about the condition of many American women today, whose efforts toward healing are really attempts to reclaim their power in a subtly but insidiously male-dominated culture.

Indeed, Patt's illness is not only a metaphor for what women often suffer in what she refers to as "an authoritarian male-structured" universe, but also a manifestation of that suffering. Because, she theorizes, she grew up "unconsciously defending being a girl" while simultaneously adopting a silent, ascending hatred for "female" qualities, she ultimately became complicit in her own sickness, as so many women do: by turning that self-hatred inward.

Because of Lind-Kyle's extensive background in the sciences, in teaching, in psychology, and in communications, she is the ideal messenger. She simply and thoroughly documents not only her story, but also, her comprehensive search for herself, for a cure, and for reason. The reader will emerge with a mutli-layered understanding of Chronic Fatigue syndrome, but also, of a plethora of treatment modalities, alternative medicines, spiritual tools, and socio-historical insights into the female condition. The texture alone of this work is worth reading.

The most profound message of this piece for me was its constant theme about the stress of losing—or never attaining—a personal power or sense of control. Over and over again the reader will encounter bits of control-slippage in her story: "I was being forced to go into the quietness" she writes in one passage; "The panic and terror of losing total control of my life. .. was horrifying," she says "in every single facet of my life to a new authority, Chronic Fatigue Immune Dysfunction Syndrome." Compensating for her low self-worth, by performing competently but ultimately, she believes, this only "diminished (her) voice as a woman," succumbing to an autoimmune disorders and immune disorders — CFIDS — was another way in which her low self-worth expressed itself: an autoimmune disease is, after all, the self attacking the self.

I believe this work is useful to anyone who suffers from or knows and loves a suffer of CFIDS. It is also invaluable to any person who might see pieces of her own story in this account. The road to empowerment just may be, for many of us, learning to recognize that our bodies will tell us what our minds may not be willing to confess: that our entire being is dependent upon our autonomy and self-esteem. It is hoped that this recounting inspires each reader to find her own voice and to sing loudly and proudly, in good health.

Laurie Wimmer, April 1992
Executive Director,
Oregon Commission for Women

INTRODUCTION

A Native American Myth

Once, on a beautiful, clear, warm, sunny day a little duckling was enjoying a wonderful morning swim on a deep, blue lake. As she gleefully swam around delighting in all the beauty there was to see, suddenly she noticed a whirling, big, black hole on the other side of the lake. This hole was way beyond the reflection of the sacred mountain.

"What is it?" she thought, "What is in the hole? What is it for?" As she swam over to investigate, she heard the wings of Mr. Dragonfly coming closer and closer.

"Where are you going?" said Mr. Dragonfly.

"Oh I am going to explore the big, black hole," said the ugly duckling.

"You can't go without my permission, I am the gate keeper."

"Oh, Mr. Dragonfly," she responded, "please, please, can I go?"

"Well, only if you keep three promises," he said.

"I will, I will. What are they?"

"You must listen to all you are told, let go of all you hold dear, and follow what the future tells you." Just before the duckling could answer, she quickly vanished into the big, black hole.

Sometime later Mr. Dragonfly was taking his morning flight over the lake. He looked down, and he couldn't believe his eyes. Swimming on the lake was a most magnificent, beautiful, graceful, white, long necked swan. He swooped down for a closer look and said,

"Who are you?"

"Oh, don't you remember me Mr. Dragonfly? I was the ugly duckling." "What happened to you?" said Mr. Dragonfly.

"Well, I did everything you told me, I listened and marveled at the future, and I gave everything up. For all of that, I was touched and sanctified by the Great Spirit. But the most important thing of all Mr. Dragonfly, is that I have been eternally blessed with the power of self-transformation."

● ● ● ● ● ● ● ● ● ● ● ● ●

WHEN SLEEPING BEAUTY WAKES UP

A Woman's Tale of the Healing of the Immune System and the Awakening of the Feminine.

Life is like a puzzle. You go about the business of living, day by day experiencing life as though you were placing events within an unknown puzzle. Only upon looking back can you see how well each piece fits so perfectly together.

This is a story of the journey that took me deep into the dark hole of a new disease called Chronic Fatigue Immune Dysfunction Syndrome. Chronic Fatigue Immune Dysfunction Syndrome or CFIDS was the catalyst that coerced me into a voyage of self discovery. It significantly reshaped my life. As I began to awaken from the deep sleep of this illness and move toward recovery, I realized that I was not only physically waking up, but that the illness was a powerful force transforming me psychologically, spiritually, and physically.

Throughout the several years of my illness the core questions I was forced to confront included: "Do I grow or do I die?" "Will I choose to live?" Illness can be either a teacher or a destroyer. When I finally chose to be taught, the healing process began to unfold like a lovely flower, or the remembering of an ancient story. The flower unfolded slowly and the ancient story of life was revealed a little at a time.

Paradoxically, in the beginning I was beyond any conscious understanding of my healing process. I became so deathly ill from CFIDS that it seemed I was actually asleep for more than three years. On the other hand, the illness awakened me to unknown parts of myself. There were times that I would ask, "Is life worth the recovery?" "Do I really want to live?" I hope my experience living with, and finally conquering Chronic Fatigue Immune Dysfunction Syndrome can be a guide and an inspiration for you to seize the opportunities offered by any devastating illness or circumstance. I will also share new insights into the old wisdoms of womanhood that came to me during the darkest moments and during the final phases of the healing. During those dark moments of my illness the "wicked witch" appeared in the guise of a number of unresolved unconscious issues in my life. I believe now that illness arises out of one's total life condition. As buried feelings begin to surface, these emotions can be a destructive tirade of hate against oneself. Mired deeply into the disease, it is difficult, however, to decipher what is real and what is not real. But with time, insight, and new skills, one can unravel the origins and deeper meaning of an illness.

CFIDS is a new disease, discovered six years ago, and as yet I have not read any personal accounts of other CFIDS healing journeys. This disease is so obscure that there is no insurance coverage, limited medical knowledge, and no traditional treatments. I have often wondered, how others have coped with CFIDS. Is their process similar to mine and how has it changed their life? During my illness, I wanted to have the opportunity to be consoled by someone who had survived the overwhelming physical and neurologic symptoms. I wanted personal assurance that I would make it. However, there was no one to talk with so I forged ahead on my own.

I knew that catastrophic illnesses or devastating situations can completely change one's life, and my illness changed me more than I was to know. At each stage of my healing, I evaluated and worked with my physical symptoms as well as with my emotional and psychological state. Each time it took me deeper into my self. As I questioned my contribution to society, my values, the domineering system I live under, and who and what I was living for, I got answers and I learned to follow them. This journey into myself was both expansive and liberating.

My first questions led to information concerning CFIDS. In Part I, "The Beginning of the Illness," I investigate the events which led to the symptoms of CFIDS. In Part II, I answer the questions, "Why am I sick and what do I have?" Although little was known about CFIDS when I contracted it, I then had to research the history and gather various medical data to give credence to my illness. In Part III, "Getting help," I offer the reader a treatment plan which is divided into three phases. A detailed description of each phase is located in Appendices A, B and C. I do not advocate that this treatment plan is the only one, but I do offer it as a model and as an inspiration to be responsible for your own wellness.

Part IV, entitled, "Journey Into Myself," is a personal description of my emotional, physical and spiritual story with CFIDS. I believe we must heal all levels of ourself. I found I went through seven states of death which were the breakdown of both my inner and outer life structures. The seven states of awakening were the experiences which shifted me to view my life differently, to feel creative and to have renewed life and energy.

Many readers may not be interested in information about CFIDS but would be interested in what I learned about the meaning of this disease. The section, "New Beginnings," explores the heart of the growing problems with women and the presence of our feminine in the world today. What led me to this exploration was a concern and a series of question I asked myself. I wondered why some professional women got sick and others did not. I questioned what happens to women's feminine side as they work in a male-dominated world. Could lifestyle change be related to the immune problems women experience? To answer these questions, I designed a research project in which I interviewed and assessed 40 professional women as to their childhood backgrounds, leadership concerns, their needs and wants and their knowledge of the feminine. The basis of this section of the book is the result of this research and some of their personal stories. These women's stories are so revealing, I have purposely held back their real names, occupations, and ages. I am convinced that immune problems will increase as we cut off our natural feminine inheritance in order to compete in the male-traditional world. Women who have immune problems are women who are dependent on, or have not taken responsibility for, their lives – and they are not in touch with their feminine.

We, as women, must raise our feminine esteem, understand our feminine image and gather our feminine knowledge by learning to trust, to stand up for each other and to bond together. Awakening this core feminine energy is done together.

> *The breezes at dawn have secrets to tell you*
> *Don't go back to sleep*
> *You must ask for what you really want*
> *Don't go back to sleep*
> *People are going back and forth*
> *Across the threshold where the two worlds touch*
> *The door is round and open*
> *Don't go back to sleep.*
>
> *Rumi- Sufi poet*

PART I

THE BEGINNING OF THE ILLNESS

Like many professional women in our society, I had struggled to be successful in my work. And like most women in our culture, I was taught to believe that getting a man was even more important. In fact, a woman could have professional success, but if she wasn't married, she was still not good enough. Perhaps you will hear echoes of your own life in my story.

In the secret place of my imagination I searched for my prince, but it took 47 years to finally find him. I had two other marriages before I found "my" Prince. Although I learned many things from these near-"Prince Charmings," neither were the right one for me. Implicit in the Cinderella story was that my prince would take care of me in all ways: emotionally, physically, mentally, and spiritually.

I met David, the man of my dreams, fifteen years before we were married and it took some doing for us to get together. He didn't just pop over and ask me to try on the glass slipper and suggest that we "live happily ever after." We were colleagues on the same college campus. I knew he was a prince of a man but I didn't know when we met that he was MY Prince. In a few years I married and, shortly after, David divorced. Eight years later I got divorced and he was still single. After we began dating, although I knew he was my real Prince, we experienced many trials of breaking up and then coming back together. I am sure Cinderella had it much easier!

The tension didn't stop after we got married. A week after our wedding, we were off to Africa, Egypt, and Cyprus for our honeymoon. Part of the trip was a consulting assignment for David. Although his pace is fast and mine is more methodical and slow, I accommodated to his pace. That was my first error in judgment. While he worked, I wrote a book about my work with learning styles. I rarely allowed myself time to let down and relax. We fed each other this hyper energy. This was my second mistake.

On our honeymoon, I remember one warm, lovely night in an outdoor cafe in Cyprus when we could have been romancing, we were deep in discussion about our plans to create a joint consulting business. Trying to match David's fast pace with my slower pace, sowed some of the seeds of my illness.

After our whirlwind honeymoon we launched into implementing our business plan. When we were colleagues on a college campus I had greatly admired David's teaching abilities and wished I could teach like him. He became my guru and I put myself in the position of student. I know now, however that to marry your "teacher" or "mentor" can really be counter-productive. For me, it not only clogged up our marriage, it also clogged up my "body works."

As we followed our business plan and started to do workshops together, I soon became frustrated with our "teacher-student" relationship. Often during my portion of the presentation, I would pause or make a mistake; David would rescue me from the situation and take over. Later, when I stated my concerns about his monopolizing the situation, David would counter that not only was I mistaken, but that he was "helping and supporting me." Since he wouldn't acknowledge the problem, we kept repeating this unhealthy pattern. My accumulated stress then increased even more and my self esteem also diminished because I was failing to be like him. I was pushing too far beyond my natural style, and, too far beyond my emotional and physical limits.

Several months later, when I completed my book, I was so exhausted that we decided to go to Hawaii for 10 days. Before we left on the trip we talked about moving from the city to the country. David's long time dream was to live in the Sierra Nevadas. I had never thought of moving away from the city. I had built my own house, as a single woman, and this gave me a feeling of worth, identity, and accomplishment. The only thing that made me even consider moving was the possibility of an earthquake, because the house was situated right on the San Andreas fault. To consider moving to the country, even for David's sake, did not inspire me.

We vacationed a week in Hawaii, and then I stayed on alone for a few extra days. During the time alone I fell into a wonderful rhythm of meditating, praying, reading, and exercising. I sat on the beach near the ocean and I began to experience the water as having tremendous power and energy. As I remained quiet and attentive, I could feel that same power and energy moving in and through me. I increasingly felt enmeshed by this energy. The longer I sat by the ocean the more I felt enthralled and captivated by its powerful presence. This was an entirely new experience.

One afternoon as the sun was setting, I noticed the breeze and the incredible force and power of the waves. With my heightened awareness, I became conscious of another presence that seemed to be behind me. But as I turned around, I saw only a large sugar cane field and one of Kauai's majestic mountains. Although I turned back to the ocean, I looked over my shoulder now and then. Was I experiencing the mountain itself? I had heard about people having a relationship with a tree or a mountain, but I never believed them. When I realized this pull toward me was actually from the mountain, however, my disquiet left and in its place was a feeling of love that tugged at my heart and emotions. The love was coming from someone or something much wiser, and much stronger, than me. Gazing at this beautiful green mountain, I felt great joy. As the sun set and I bid my mountain-lover good-bye, I sensed that it wanted me to return to the beach the same time the following day.

I came back to that same spot many times over the next several days. Each time the feelings of being loved by this powerful presence deepened and got stronger. The last time I sat there on the beach, I felt the mountain say that I was to create communities of women. I thought, "You're suggesting I do what?" But the mountain was silent. And it was time for me to return to the mainland, to David, and home.

As the plane took off the next day, we circled over my large green mountain. Tears suddenly welled up and streamed down my face; I felt as though I was leaving a lover behind. The mountain had given me a message about women that I would only understand years later. And, I wasn't to realize, until many years later, that this was the first conscious experience with my feminine self.

Soon after returning to the mainland, although I lost both the awareness and the feeling of my mountain, the deep memory of it convinced me that I was ready for a quiet country life. Now I thought I wanted to be away from traffic so that I could experience the presence of nature as I had with the mountain. A year later, we moved. But in the end it was difficult to leave, because I let go of the home that I had built and loved so much. The more my resistance to leaving grew, the more the real estate contract was filled with increased difficulties. I believed that my identity was being sold along with my worth — and my creativity; and, I was going into an unknown place. The mounting stress was beyond my emotional strength. Would the new home in the country be able to replace this sanctuary that had been such a major part of my life? I was unsure. With my therapy practice closed, and having said good-bye to my favorite spiritual women's group, David and I set off for Grass Valley, California, in the foothills of the Sierra Nevada mountains.

The house was on five acres facing a lake, with 200 acres of trees behind us that belonged to a Christian camp. There was a fifteen acre horse ranch to the south and about a fourth of a mile up the road to the north was our only neighbor. The day we arrived the roof began leaking. As the rains came, water poured through the roof, into the windows and down the walls. I left everything I had known for over 40 years for this? Not only was I again emotionally stressed to the limit, I had no idea what type of work I might do. I had not made plans for me, and my professional work. Was I going to repair leaking roofs and windows for a living? The green mountain seemed far, far away.

For the first three months I went along with David's grand scheme for us to commute and work in the Bay Area four days every week. But by the fourth month I was confused, exhausted, and very unhappy. Was I living in the country or in the city? I found it harder and harder to keep up with the hectic pace. I found myself doing strange things like walking up stairs but not knowing where I was or where I was going. Then, I would forget why I was doing something, or become irrational and emotionally upset over insignificant matters. This strange pattern of behavior, plus my general tiredness, began to concern me.

I had heard of an outstanding woman physician in the Bay Area who used a holistic approach to medicine and with her patients. I went to her for a routine examination. As she questioned me about my life situation and my health history, I broke down and sobbed. My sadness was hidden no longer. I thought that I was an emancipated woman, I had fallen into the trap that so many women do and let my husband, my "Prince Charming" make my choices for me. Since he was my prince, I believed he knew best. Plus, I rationalized, I couldn't disappoint him in any way. And, most of all, I couldn't risk losing him.

My physician suggested that I not commute for two weeks. She told me to go back to Grass Valley and decide where I wanted to live. Did I want to live in the country or back in the city? It seemed an impossible decision to make. I didn't want to stay in the country, but I couldn't afford to return to my city home. Begrudgingly, I followed my doctor's suggestion and went back to the country where everything supposedly was peaceful, and full of love. I now knew, however, that I could not find the love in the country that I had felt from my Hawaiian mountain. I felt no joy or peace. In fact, I felt awful. And, I was alone, without friends, and with no meaningful work. At least the rain had stopped but I was left very much alone during most of the week to ponder and accept the decision I had made.

At first, it was wonderful to be out of the whirl and out of the intensity of the city. But what was at first wonderful became a nightmare. Several days after I returned to Grass Valley, I became ill. I could only stay up for four hours at a stretch without having to go back to bed. I started to have night sweats. I was frightened of being alone; panic and terror would sweep through me at night. My body was in constant pain. I was highly emotional and depressed. During the day I would feel waves of unhappiness wash over me, and not know why I felt so dark and gloomy. I was afraid that I was going crazy, and that all this was in my imagination. Nothing this intensely physical and emotional had ever happened to me before.

The two weeks stretched into two months. During this time, I used the excuse that I wasn't sick, I had to manage the remodeling on the house. The workman came at 10:00 a.m. so I could sleep in. He took two hour lunches so I could sleep again in the afternoon, and then, he left by 6:30 p.m. so I could get to bed by seven in the evening. It was difficult to be professionally non-productive. When I intimated to the carpenter that I was a professional woman he would look at me like, "You've got to be kidding." I was beginning to feel like a nobody. I looked awful. I had lost weight, my face sagged, and I felt emotionally lost.

One day while browsing in a bookstore I picked up a book entitled *Are You Really Too Sensitive?* by Marcy Calhoun. As I thumbed through the pages, I read:

> *Structural ultra-sensitives will live and work in the world surviving and achieving, until a crisis surfaces in their lives and then the structure they have built for themselves will no longer work for them. They are not only inflexible in the world, they are also inflexible within their own structure. They are unwilling (or do not know how) to make the changes that would cause them to grow . . . If what you are doing is stifling or suffocating to yourself, your spiritual side will create a crisis to end the suffocating actions in your life. When you have continually said no to change that means you are going against the survival system of the body, mind, emotion, and spirit. Then your life support systems will take over for your own survival, which forces you to move no matter how painful that movement may*

> *be. It may occur either in a relationship, a career*
> *or a family situation. The painful process will*
> *make you create movement. The movement will*
> *make you realize that what you have been doing*
> *is not working and now you must face and*
> *understand your emotional side.*[1]

I was startled by Marcy's words. They sounded like my life. How could I could find out more about this structural process? I called the publisher and discovered that the author lived in a nearby town. Making an appointment to meet with her, I worked up enough energy to make the visit. She immediately told me I was very sick and that if I hadn't moved to the country I would probably have died. It was her opinion that I needed to be in a relaxing environment of the country. She also said I needed lots of oxygen and to take deep breaths. Marcy also told me I would go through the "Dark Night of The Soul." Although I had heard this phrase before, I really didn't know what she was talking about. I was soon to find out.

Two months after my visit to Marcy, my doctor told me that I had a severe case of Epstein-Barr virus. I resisted the fact that I was sick but a wide variety of puzzling physical symptoms continued to surface. I began to have debilitating stiffness in my joints, shoulders, and hips. A tightness in my throat seemed to be connected to my stomach. I had a constant, gnawing flu-like tiredness. I was continually sleepy and wanted to stay in bed all the time. I began to forget simple things like taking my vitamins; I put the eggs in the freezer. I walked down by the lake and suddenly forgot which leg to put down. Thoroughly frightened, I lost balance and fell down.

David was busy commuting and working so he didn't see many of my worst incidents. When at home he noticed some of the unusual behaviors and would ask me about them, but he seemed mostly un-concerned. And at first, I thought that I could be going through menopause. Then, I rationalized that being miles away from people might be the cause. As I took walks around the lake I told myself that with all the beauty of the country, and, being away from the noise and traffic, I *should* be contented and joyful. Instead, my surroundings only made me realize how lonely I was. I felt dead. I literally thought my life was over. I saw no way out.

I telephoned Marcy for some more advice, but because of her busy traveling schedule we were unable to get together. She suggested that I see one of her colleagues. When I met with this woman, she suggested that I needed to make changes in my life because I was not getting my needs met. Because I didn't want to hear this, I responded angrily. I was in denial and very defensive. Besides, what could I do? I couldn't move back to the city. It was too expensive, and my prince was extremely happy living in the country. I could sense that David couldn't wait to come home. But summer was coming on and I was getting weaker and weaker. The heat of the day failed to cool at night and all my energy was drained by it. So I was stuck in the house, alone most of the time, feeling exhausted and deeply confused.

Finally, I returned to my doctor and was told the blood test results showed that I had a severe case of the Epstein-Barr virus. The doctor explained that it was a herpes-like virus that causes infectious mononucleosis and is associated with Burkitt's lymphoma and nasopharyngeal carcinoma, a cancer of the soft palate. The doctor told me that there were no medications that she could recommend for the condition and the only thing to do was rest. And eat healthy food.

Well, that confirmed it. I actually had an identifiable illness. I went home and to bed! The response of my friends to my illness was very disappointing. They would say to me, "You look fine, and you sound fine. What's your problem?" Most people knew little or nothing about the Epstein-Barr virus. In fact, after a while most of my friends began to distance themselves. I discovered that chronic disease victims are usually forgotten or ignored after the initial acute stage of an illness.

One of the most difficult responses for me to handle was from my spiritual friends. They suggested that if we indeed create our own reality, then how was I making myself sick? I, therefore, "must be at fault, and if I would simply take responsibility, then I would get better." This concept, however is very hard to manage at the initial stages of a debilitating illness such as the Epstein-Barr virus. My immune system was weakened and the virus had surfaced. In the swamp of my depression, these indictments from friends only made my symptoms worse. In principle, I valued the concept of self-creating responsibility, but, as yet, I didn't know how to use it to help me regain my health. The healing process would begin later. I had yet to reach the depths of the darker side of my illness. There were more lessons to be learned.

As I sank deeper into depression, a call from a former client gave me some hope. She told me about a woman who had been "asleep" with EBV for five years. When I called this woman she give me some advice and perspective about the seriousness of my condition. First, she recommend that I have someone take care of me. She told me about the intense emotional swings that I would have, and that I would start inflammatory arguments with David that would be dangerous for our relationship. She further cautioned me that I might put much of the blame for my illness on him.

Another valuable piece of advice was her dietary recommendation. She emphasized that I should use no sugar, no caffeine, no alcohol, or any dairy products. She suggested that I have a high daily intake of protein and low fat intake. Her helpful advice and suggestions gave me some structure to follow and also provided a feeling that I wasn't alone. Even though she had given me practical advice, I was still a bit discouraged as to my prospect for the future. I couldn't believe this woman had already struggled for over five years. I was frightened at the thought that I had years of this illness still ahead of me.

David then called his daughter, Shellie, to come and take care of me for a few weeks. Finally, a sense of relief came over me. I needed the attention and acknowledgment of my illness along with some practical help. Fortunately, Shellie was very special and caring and being with her helped my spirit. Her daily nurturing allowed me to let go to the seriousness of my situation. And, I came face to face with the question of how I was going to survive financially. All my life, I had been self-sufficient. Was I going to allow myself to be dependent on someone else? I enjoyed teaching and counseling and now I lacked the energy to do either one. I also saw my husband creating a new business and living the life style I thought I wanted. He was advancing, while I was standing still.

I looked out the window at the horse pasture and I felt that I had literally been put out to pasture. I hated seeing life pass me by. I became increasingly sad and anything slightly emotional I would tend to amplify. I felt like a mental case. I was a bundle of emotions strung way out of control.

Although other people helped to care for me after Shellie went back to school, I was still unable to cope with noise, extra people, or out of the ordinary events. Beyond the practical care giving, my change in diet was essential to feeling better. Learning that protein was critical, I ate meat or fish for breakfast, lunch, and dinner. Food and a great deal of sleep were primary factors in beginning the healing process. I began to sleep all night without waking. But I still had the aching, tightness in my throat and the upset stomach. I would have breakfast in the morning, then sleep till noon. I ate lunch and then slept until around 5 o'clock. I would then have dinner and go to bed for the night. I was unable to concentrate well enough to listen to music, watch TV, read a book, or meditate. I lacked the energy to exercise. Yet, I remembered Marcy telling me that I needed oxygen. How was I going to get oxygen if I couldn't exercise? At this point, I didn't know that exercise actually made the illness worse. I was simply trying to survive each day and cope with my feelings of being inadequate and worthless.

PART II

WHAT DO I HAVE? WHY AM I SO SICK?

Beginning on June 9, 1987, the following physical and psychological symptoms forced me to evaluate my health and clearly admit that my physical and emotional condition was deteriorating.

Physical Symptoms
1. A slight temperature and malaise
2. Low energy along with a feeling of exhaustion
3. Body tiredness even after a night's sleep
4. Constriction, pressure, and tightness in my throat
5. A pulling sensation on the lower half of my face, with nerves that were vibrating and tingling
6. An empty feeling in my stomach and soreness in my gastro-intestinal area; pain in the right side of my abdomen
7. My shoulders, arms, and hip joints were extremely sore and achy
8. Loss of coordination and balance
9. Swollen fingers
10. Night sweats
11. Interrupted sleep
12. Dizziness
13. Nausea
14. Glandular swelling
15. Generalized body weakness

Psychological Symptoms
1. Overwhelming feeling of depression
2. Loss of memory
3. Inability to concentrate on conversation or simple tasks

4. Anxiety and fear without knowing the source
5. Over-reaction to minimal stress situations; highly emotional behavior that was not warranted by the circumstance
6. Anti-social behavior expressed without warning to whomever was with me
7. Lethargy and lack of responsiveness to normal daily activity

Most of my symptoms were classic signs of what is known now as Chronic Fatigue Immune Dysfunction Syndrome. I was diagnosed, however, as having Epstein-Barr virus. The EBV serology blood test I was given measures the presence of antibodies to the Epstein-Barr virus. Actually there is controversy among physicians as to whether or not this blood test is useful in diagnosing EBV. Some doctors have found that not all patients who have EBV will show abnormal counts of the antibodies in the test results. There also seems to be no correlation between test results and presence of symptoms for many people. The reason is that many EBV patients also have positive results when testing for other diseases, such as measles. However, the results of my test showed a high "titer" count in my blood. I now have found that a "high titer" does not necessarily indicate current viral replication. But my doctor did not question the results of the test because of the broad range of my physical and psychological symptoms.

As friends heard about my illness, they began to send me newspaper articles about the new "Yuppie Disease," Epstein-Barr virus. I appreciated the thought, but I didn't appreciate the insinuating remarks intimating that I was in the yuppie whirl. The newspaper articles repeatedly said that physically active, highly creative and responsible women between the ages of 27-40 were affected. Because I had just turned 50, I asked myself, "Why me?" And, apart from the affirmation and support of my own doctor and the EBV test, it seemed that many in the medical community were not taking EBV seriously. As I read the articles and felt the misunderstanding of some friends, I began to doubt myself. At times I began to think I would never be vibrant and healthy again. Was this all in my head? Where was my beautiful green mountain?

As the months went by I had minimal contact with others who had been diagnosed with EBV. Talking with a few EBV patients, I felt better knowing I was not alone, but I would often feel depressed after a conversation focused on "poor me" and "Oh, I am such a victim." Although we needed each other to compare notes, I still was in denial we were ill and couldn't face what was happening to my life. The conversations exhausted me; for the sake of my own survival I discontinued direct contact with EBV patients. This, of course, left me even more alone.

From reading medical journal articles, I now understood that the virus EBV was always present in the body. I became hopeful when I understood that the symptoms would eventually diminish if I took good care of myself. But the virus itself would remain. When the symptoms vanished this indicated that the virus was simply inactive until reactivated. Finally, the one ray of light I had was the desire to find out more about this disease. In 1988 I began to question. Just what is this Epstein-Barr virus? How does it relate to mononucleosis? What was the relationship to the HIV virus and AIDS as some articles suggested?

What were the preventive measures that could stop the illness from occurring? How did one get it? And was there any cure? To begin answering these questions I first had to gain a depth of understanding about the virus.

What Is A Virus?

The virus is the smallest known type of infectious organism. Viral infections range from the trivial and harmless such as warts, the common cold, and other minor respiratory tract infections, to extremely serious diseases, such as rabies, AIDS and probably some types of cancer. The structure of a single virus particle (called a virion) consists simply of an inner core of nucleic acid surrounded by one or two protective shells (called capsids) made of protein. The nucleic acid at the core of the virus consists of a string of genes that contains coded instructions for making copies of the virus.

A virus is parasitic and its sole activity is to invade cells of other organisms to make copies of themselves. A virus uses mammalian cell tissue because it cannot live outside living cells. Outside live tissue it is inert and lacks independent metabolism. Because of its parasitic nature a virus only replicates within a living host cell. When the virus invades the nucleus of the host cells it may not at first replicate itself, but rather it may "hide" in the cell, sometimes becoming reactivated months or years later. So when the doctor said to me that the symptoms could go away, but the virus was still in me I began to realize that in response to certain triggering events, the virus could be reactivated and produce another round of the same symptoms I had.

I further discovered that viruses can enter the body in a variety of ways. They could be inhaled in droplets of fluid, swallowed in food and liquids, passed through punctured skin in the saliva of feeding insects or rabid dogs, accidentally transmitted on the needles of tattooists or intravenous drug users, or simply when someone got their ears pierced. No single virus shows all of these transmission modes. One could get a virus from a doctor during an examination, or in the mucus membranes of the genital tract during sexual intercourse, or be contaminated in the conjunctiva of the eye. We know so little medically about viruses that there are probably many other ways that we contract them. I learned that there were 12 known viral groups, and that each virus has different strategies of making copies of itself after invading the host body cell tissue.

What Is Epstein-Barr Virus?

At one time or another, most everyone is exposed to the Epstein-Barr virus, EBV. In fact, the infection with this virus is so common that 90 percent of the adult population of the U.S. over the age of thirty has been infected. Epstein-Barr virus is a member of the herpes family of viruses, which also includes herpes simplex 1 and 2. Simplex 1 causes oral herpes, creating cold sores. Simplex 2 is responsible for genital herpes. The varicella-zoster virus causes chicken pox and shingles. The cytomegalovirus causes an illness similar to mononucleosis. There is a new herpes virus called human herpes virus 6. It is thought that HHV6 may cause diseases similar to those caused by the Epstein-Barr virus. EBV has been associated to two cancers: Burkitt's lymphoma and nasopharyngeal carcinoma, affecting the pharynx above the soft palate.

The Epstein-Barr virus plays havoc with our immune system. The immune system is our interface with the environment and also our defense system against infection. This system has two basic functions. First, to recognize anything that may be detrimental to our health, and, then, to respond in some protective way. The immune system is composed of the tonsils, adenoids, thymus gland, the lymph nodes throughout the body, the bone marrow, the white blood cells, other cells in the lymphatic system, the spleen, the appendix, and patches of lymphoid tissue in the intestinal tract. This clever system not only protects against infections but is able to distinguish what is organically us and the various fluids circulating through our bodies, and to identify something from the outside that is not part of our organic system. The immune system also recognizes and takes appropriate action against those materials that ought not to be in the body, including abnormal and damaging components. For example, it can seek out and destroy diseased cells infected by germs, as well as recognize and destroy tumor cells. The immune system also prevents the body's own cells from coming under attack by the immune system. There is, however, a condition that is called autoimmunity, when the immune system mistakenly attacks the body's own tissues. Examples of autoimmune diseases are rheumatoid arthritis, rheumatic fever, lupus, thyroditis, multiple sclerosis, type I diabetes, and ulcerative colitis. Autoimmune reactions may be set off by infected tissue, an injury to the body or emotional trauma.

The EBV sets up residence in white blood cells, called the B-type lymphocytes. Lymphocytes are formed in the lymph glands rather than in the bone morrow. These cells roam freely around between the blood stream and the lymph glands. The B cells manufacture Y-shaped antibodies and have very specific receptor sites on their surface. This structure allows the B cells to recognize and attack a particular virus. These specific antibodies fit into one particular virus the way a key fits into one particular lock. If the key is not engineered for that lock it will not work. This specificity serves two purposes. First, it ensures that these antibodies will attack only foreign antigens and not the cells of the body. These specific antibodies also serve as a memory, allowing the immune system to remember a specific infectious agent. When the infection is over, the immune system retains these specific antibodies. If that particular strain of virus should ever invade the body again, the immune system will be able to respond quickly and powerfully, preventing a recurrence of that illness. The B lymphocyte cells also produce another class of antibodies that when combined with nine specialized proteins can achieve that same effect. These proteins, called complement proteins, circulate throughout the blood, and are lethal toxins that do not have the safeguard of specificity that antibodies do. These proteins destroy any cell they come in contact with. Our B cells are a fail-safe system to protect the body from these deadly proteins. Also the B-type cells are regulated and given orders by the T-type lymphocyte cell.

The T-type lymphocytes are responsible for hypersensitivity situations, such as allergies. That means antibodies are formed against harmless substances because T-cells have mistaken and misread them as potentially harmful. So, when there is a problem with the T-type lymphocytes, B cells, whose role it is to protect us from secondary attacks by forming antibodies, will also be affected. As I began to understand more about EBV, and about viruses in general, I wanted to understand more about the relationship of EBV to mononucleosis and also its possible connection to AIDS.

Is EBV Related To Mononucleosis?

Mononucleosis and EBV have many similar features, particularly the symptom of fatigue. Infectious mononucleosis is caused either by the Epstein-Barr virus or by cytomegalovirus, both members of the herpesvirus family. But the two are different in that EBV tends not to produce high fevers, an enlarged liver or spleen, and major changes in blood count. Mononucleosis has been called "the kissing disease" because of this infection though saliva from another person. Some people think that Epstein-Barr virus is also spread through saliva, but EBV can also be spread through blood transfusions.

How Does EBV Relate to AIDS?

Is there a connection between EBV and AIDS? AIDS is a deficiency of the immune system due to infection with the human immunodeficiency virus, HIV, involving the T4 lymphocytes. As HIV enters into a cell it not only multiples but changes the genetic code within that cell. Normally the DNA (which is deoxyribonucleic acid found in cells to encode instructions for building cells, tissues, and organs through the manufacture of specific proteins) makes RNA— ribonucleic acid—which carries an activated amino acid and participates in the manufacture of a protein molecule.

In the case of AIDS, the virus HIV is a RNA retrovirus that reverses the usual sequence by which genetic information is passed through the body. The retrovirus makes an enzyme called reverse transcriptase which makes a mirror image of itself. The mirrored image then incorporates itself into the DNA where it makes copies of itself similar to the way a computer saves information on a magnetic disk in order to make a permanent record of it. At the core of the cell tissue, then, is a bundle of the HIV-infected RNA. This is like having a virus in the computer, which eventually begins to eat up the existing information in the computer. The virus, in essence, is recreating the code of life, but is ironically spreading death through the very process by which life is conceived. The new DNA becomes part of the host cell and countless infected RNA copies emerge, wrapping themselves in protein, streaming out into the blood, and spreading to every part of the body.

When this organism is multiplying rapidly, a person ends up with his or her own personal strain of the AIDS virus. Even though the antibodies of our immune system may wipe out millions of the AIDS viruses another more resistant AIDS strain will mutate and repopulate the blood.

What the researchers tell us is that the virus then may change and mutate again and again. Because of this mutability of the AIDS virus, it is next to impossible to develop a vaccine that could stimulate a universally protective antibody response. As the immune system loses hold, even organisms that normally do not invade a human cell begin to do so, initiating new diseases. Researchers have recently identified a retrovirus fragment in Chronic Fatigue Immune Dysfunction Syndrome patients. More testing needs to be done to verify that this retrovirus plays a significant role in this disease. CFIDS by its name indicates an immune *dysfunction* and AIDS indicates an immune *deficiency*.

Why Are There No Definitive Tests, Prevention, Or Cure For Chronic Fatigue Syndrome?

I began to talk with people and read as much as I could about the history of CFIDS. I wanted to find out how the disease evolved, and why so little information was available. I soon learned that the first publicized exposure to what would eventually be called Chronic Fatigue Syndrome, occurred in a small Nevada town near Lake Tahoe.

In 1984 Drs. Paul Cheney and Daniel Peterson began to see an unusually large number of extremely fatigued patients in their private practices in Incline Village, Nevada. These patients had flu-like symptoms that just didn't go away. In January 1985, Dr. James Jones wrote an article "Evidence for Active Epstein-Barr Virus (EBV) Infection in Patients with Persistent, Unexplained Illness," published in the *Annals of Internal Medicine*. He studied patients with symptoms similar to mine and came to the conclusion that the cause of the symptoms may be associated with recognizable illnesses other than infectious mononucleosis.

At the same time, in 1985, three hundred of the 30,000 residents of the resort communities of Incline Village, Tahoe City, and Truckee, Nevada, became ill with a continuous flu. Drs. Peterson and Cheney began to suspect that reactivated Epstein-Barr virus (EBV) might be responsible for this flu-like illness. They reported this epidemic to both public and governmental health agencies. Their reports to the press so enraged the town leaders of Incline Village, however, they started a smear campaign against the two doctors in order to run them out of town. The fear of town leaders was that tourists and their dollars would stay away from the resort and hurt business profits if the public heard about the new disease. Because of this smear campaign, one doctor, Dr. Paul Cheney, relocated in North Carolina. In 1986, *Science* magazine published information that a newly discovered Human B-lymphotropic virus (HBLV) had been found. The article suggested that HBLV was a possible cause of Chronic Fatigue Syndrome. This new virus had been isolated from AIDS patients at the National Cancer Institute.

The authors of other medical journal articles stated that EBV could be a cofactor to another virus. In other words, there could be more than one virus involved. In this scenario two viruses would be acting synergistically, flourishing together where neither could manage alone. The research articles asserted that EBV is activated when the cells are invaded by human B-lymphotropic virus, HBLV, (AIDS is HTLV). This action impairs the normal functions of B cells but also stimulates the latent viruses to become more active. Because of this new information indicating that EBV was just one of several viruses working together, the name of this symptom complex was changed to Chronic Fatigue Immune Dysfunction Syndrome, CFIDS.

Can It Be Transmitted?

As I followed the research into CFIDS, I received conflicting views on how the disease is actually transmitted. A critical question for me was whether I could transmit the disease to David or to my family and friends. My understanding at the time, 1987, was that the virus was somehow latent in the cells of the person and that some environmental, physical, or psychological condition activated it in the individual. This view holds that everyone has this virus; some of us are activating it in some way. The recent discovery that CFIDS is possibly a retrovirus like AIDS indicates that there may be a blood transmission process, as well as other possible transmission means to spread the disease.

Another question I had was whether CFIDS typically progressed to another disease? I had heard of no individual dying of it. I had heard, however, of many who ended their own lives from the overwhelming depression the disease created. And, in my own experience, I believed that I was progressively getting weaker, psychologically and physically. I, learned, too, that with a defective immune system I would be open to various types of secondary infection. So, my reasoning at that time was that it could possibly be progressive to other diseases. Later, I learned that CFIDS would affect brain cells as well as the thyroid and adrenal glands.

The Psychological Dynamics Of CFIDS

After the diagnosis of having the Epstein-Barr virus and trying to understand, medically, what this disease was all about, a new dynamic entered my life.

Throughout this first phase of the illness, I had resigned myself to being sick, alone, and unproductive. But within six months after the diagnosis I started to feel better. As I emerged from my mental and emotional grogginess, two factors emerged clearly, out of the fog: I was living David's dream and he was living mine. For 20 years he had longed to live in the Sierra Nevada mountains. And now with a home in his beloved mountains, he was creating a new business located three and half hours away in the San Francisco Bay Area. And, I, the one who dreamed and talked of being in the city, was stuck in some God-forsaken place in the foothills of the Sierra Nevadas, sick in bed. Something was wrong. I was either saying good bye to David as he drove off into the sunset, or anxiously waiting for his home-coming. When he arrived home, however, he was often glued to the phone talking to clients or to his office staff, even while eating dinner. Deep disappointment and anger surfaced from within me.

I knew I wasn't the most energetic, happy, or physically healthy person to be around, but I also knew that I didn't like what was happening to our relationship. So in December 1987 I confronted this unhappy turn of events. I told David that if he remained away from me both mentally and physically, then I didn't want to be with him. I accused him of purposefully creating a life that was causing my illness. "What kind of life is this to make me stay alone all the time while you are with people and being productive?" My words were hard and hurtful. I was angry and I wanted to make David feel my pain and struggle. I no longer could tolerate the unhealthy existence I was living. I worked myself into a frenzy that touched every wounded place in his soul. In my emotional and physical state, all I could think of to solve the situation was to separate and move out. This shocked David deeply. Although I craved attention and needed nurturing, he was preoccupied with keeping the business going. I later discovered that these highly emotional responses of depression, anger, and irrational behavior are some of the psychological symptoms of CFIDS.

I tell this part of my story because many who are in the

acute stages of CFIDS often lose their relationships through irrational behavior. The loss of friends, spouse, or lover and even children, can result in more stress causing the illness to get worse. CFIDS patients have a host of neurological problems; research indicates that there is a reduction of blood flow to parts of the brain which may be the cause of memory loss and a wide range of emotional and personality swings. In some cases, deeply hidden anger and rage that have been suppressed suddenly explode in unexpected and uncontrolled ways.

My personal experience with CFIDS is not unusual; I have heard over and over again that individuals with this disease have difficulty keeping both casual and intimate relationships together. If a relationship is not strong enough to handle the ill person's anger and rage, it will often fall apart and dissolve. The increasing tragedy is that many CFIDS patients end up living by themselves because of broken and battered relationships. There is then guilt, pain, and deep remorse for the grief they feel they have caused loved ones. Even when they try to resolve the dilemma, the same angry pattern is often repeated with another person.

Within the irony of this forced isolation, however, is my belief that this separation from people is what CFIDS patients need for a period of time. They need to be alone in order to restore, reduce the stress, center in on themselves, and begin to listen to their bodies and to the inner voice. This dilemma hit a deep chord in me. I was hurt that I wasn't being taking care of and being nurtured. I was brutally angry with David, with others around me, and with this disease for limiting and destroying my life. On the other hand, I wanted to take care of myself by being out in the world working.

My explosive announcement to separate set David in a whirl of reflection and concern about our lives. Fortunately, he also had become aware that his work was too consuming. He also felt out of touch with himself. After many long and arduous discussions between us, David made a major decision to leave the company in San Francisco and return to his private consulting practice. I had won! I was beginning to get my needs met, and as a result I soon began to feel better. When David chose us rather than the business, his decision relieved the stress and pressure on me. My depression and fatigue went away and I felt like myself for the first time in over two years. It was the first Christmas with family and friends in our new home. Pleased with the change, I felt so much physically and emotionally better that I went back to my old diet, and I was able to keep pace with the holiday cooking, eating, entertaining, and other festivities.

In January with my energy almost back to normal, David and I decided to do a few workshops with clients, together. I knew David would have to carry most of the load but, because I helped create them, I wanted to participate and lead the workshops as much as possible. After the first workshop, however, I noticed that I was not altogether back to normal but, because I was feeling much better than before, we did a few more. Then, in April 1988 all the symptoms appeared again. I couldn't stay awake and I was losing energy very rapidly. It was the beginning of a CFIDS relapse.

My energy level was worse than it had been the first time. I could barely get out of bed or talk. I stayed in bed much more during the day and could do less and less around the house. I had no stamina and the depression that enveloped me was devastating. I saw no reason to live. In this condition I didn't want to be alive. For the first time in my life I actually believed that I was going to die. I began to let go of people and of things around me and gave up on trying to get well.

When David would leave for a few days to work, I found I couldn't stand to be alone. On one of his five days away I sank deeper and deeper into depression. On the fourth day alone, deep into the darkness, a friend telephoned; I could barely speak a coherent sentence. She telephoned some other friends, and they came and collected me and took me to their home. Being with them didn't change my feelings of depression and loneliness, however. No matter where I was, with or without others, I felt isolated and alone. This feeling of aloneness was so devastating that I went into a deeper slump.

One of my women friends said a friend of hers got so sick that she was confined to a wheel chair. Her husband then left her for another woman. With that piece of information my fear and guilt increased intensely, and I dropped even lower into my depression. Then she encouraged me to read an article written by another women who had been seriously ill. The article, she said, described this woman's experience of illness as a means of bringing her to a spiritual awakening.

The article explained that the duration of her illness facilitated an unraveling of all the things that kept her from her spiritual self and from finding contact with her soul. The emotional instability and physical illness the author described sounded quite familiar to the symptoms and behaviors I had been experiencing. This article piqued my interest because the woman also described that the relationship with her partner had been strengthened rather than weakened through those trying times. Her uplifting story encouraged me to ponder the possibility that maybe I was here for some reason and perhaps my life had not lost its deeper meaning. Was my Hawaiian mountain trying to communicate with me? Out of aloneness and out of one of the darkest passages of my life, a question slowly formed. "Could something be developing on an inner level within me of which I was not aware?"

This awareness that perhaps my illness had some deeper meaning, raised my energy level enough to help me find a doctor who had knowledge of CFIDS. It had been a whole year since I had seen my M.D. in the city. Surely, I thought, the medical community must know more about the disease and have some kind of medication to prescribe. Most offices I telephoned, however, said they didn't work with my kind of problem. Others offices said that they had a full patient load, and didn't have room for a new patient. Finally, one doctor nearby said I could have an appointment in three weeks.

While waiting for the doctor in the reception area, I became so weak I could no longer even sit in a chair. I waited for my appointment lying on a gurney. After telling the doctor my story, he told David and me that there was really nothing he could do other than prescribe the diet I was on already and give me biweekly B-12 shots. Then he said, "Come back in two weeks." And I said, "Why? I just hope I will be alive in two weeks." The doctor suggested that David get into some kind of therapy to help support him through my illness. He said that most marriages fail when one of the partners has a chronic illness. The doctor's encouragement and suggestion was a blessing for our marriage and our relationship. David reported later that his private sessions with a therapist, gave him perspective and helped him balance the pressure and tensions from my illness.

After the visit to the country doctor another enormous depression hit me; I believed there was no where else to get help. This doctor was my last hope and only resource and I knew that what he was doing was not aggressive enough to really turn this illness around. I hit an all time low and felt like I would simply die and turn to dust. Although David was away attending his daughter's graduation, he sensed the seriousness of my situation; he called every two hours to make sure I was still alive. There is no doubt in my mind that the individuals who die from CFIDS are those who commit suicide. The depression pulls so hard that it seems like ending your life is the only solution to relieve the misery. But, it was here at the darkest time, at the lowest ebb of my life, that something inside shifted. Amazingly, out of nowhere, I received a surge of vibrant energy from the Universe.

Just after this powerful mental, emotional, and spiritual shift two events happened. First I received from several different sources, information about a clinic just an hour's drive from our home that treated EBV patients. A physician there combined both the traditional and alternative methods of healing.

The second occurrence was that in May, 1988, Dr. Paul Cheney (one of the doctors in Incline Village, Nevada, who was now doing research on CFIDS) announced an apparent rise in cases both in the U.S. and overseas, suggesting that there was now a pandemic increase of the disease. Another publication also stated that there was a marked recognition by the medical community of the diagnosis of a new disease, officially called Chronic Fatigue Immune Deficiency Syndrome. The list of symptoms which defined a typical CFIDS case matched my own symptoms. It seems strange to confess this fact, but I was actually glad to have a definable disease. After being treated and thinking of myself as some crazy woman for so long, I felt much better about myself. I told my friends that the medical authorities even gave my illness a new name; I had a legitimate disease, CFIDS.

The diagnostic criteria are developed from a surveillance study at the Center of Disease Control in Atlanta, Georgia. The list of symptoms are ranked in the order of frequency as reported to the medical community. You can notice the degree to which any of these symptoms may be affecting you. If you have felt confused about what is happening, take heart — you are not a crazy, deranged person. Possibly the awareness of these symptoms will give you some perspective on a treatment process.

Physical Symptoms, Chronic Fatigue Immune Dysfunction Syndrome, CFIDS

1. Fatigue — persists for at least 6 months, will occur after minimal exercise
2. Flu-like symptoms
3. Sleep disturbance — lasts for at least 6 months
4. Muscle weakness
5. Strong headaches
6. Muscle pains
7. Sore throats
8. Joint pains
9. Painful lymph nodes
10. Frequent fevers

Neuro-Psychological Symptoms, CFIDS

1. Mild depression
2. Inability to concentrate
3. Forgetfulness
4. Excessive irritability
5. Photophobia — eyes hurting from sunlight and overhead ultraviolet lights.
6. Mental confusion about simple decision-making.
7. Geometric forms of light constantly moving in the eyes.

PART III

GETTING HELP

Phase I Of My Treatment

Out of the blue, I received three telephone calls about the Preventive Medical Clinic located in Sacramento, California. One caller informed me that the clinic treated CFIDS patients by giving them hydrogen peroxide drips into their veins. Other callers told me about the clinic's food allergy testing and about a man's recovery from CFIDS.

When I called for an appointment I asked to talk with someone about the clinic and how it worked. I learned that the clinic used alternative therapies to help patients regain optimal health. Alternative therapies have a different outlook on health from that viewed by traditional orthodox medicine. Traditional medical practitioners of allopathic medicine tend to think of the body as a machine, and they treat the broken parts of the machine like a mechanic does. In this sense, they treat the diseased parts of the body and not the total patient. Alternative, or holistic practitioners, like to think of the patient as a whole unit composed of mind, body, and spirit. They often view illness as an outward physical reflection of an internal mental, emotional, or spiritual problem. They work to treat the problem at its roots in the patient's body as well as in the inner self. This alternative clinic was a combination of both traditional allopathic and alternative holistic type practices and treatments.

I was pleased to find that the clinic was directed by a medical doctor, but that the clinic also had a staff that included a chiropractor, biochemist, homeopath, massage therapist, acupuncturist, psychologist, and nutritionist. The clinic used allergy testing, cardiovascular monitoring, chelation and I.V. therapies, colon hydro-therapy, and had a clinical laboratory for diagnosing blood, urine and feces. There also was a nutritional center for bulk organic foods, herbs, supplements, books and literature on health, and a restaurant serving organic meals.

I went through a comprehensive testing process which included blood, urine, and feces panels. Thermography, a test which reveals temperature ranges within the body (this test provides an accurate picture of circulation in body surface areas); an E.K.G; the Heidelberg gastric analysis (an evaluation of the stomach pH and digestive ability), and the treadmill stress testing.

My diagnosis from this whole battery of tests indicated that I had Hashimoto's thyroditis, anemia, arthritis, gastritis, Epstein-Barr virus, and Candida. Now that I look back I wonder if I had all of these things. I knew I was very sick and I was not at all surprised with all the other conditions that were identified. I felt that the clinic had been thorough and I knew they were on the right track.

After reviewing the test results with the doctor, a specific treatment plan was prescribed for me. I followed the first phase of the treatment plan from July 1988 to December 1988.

PHASE I TREATMENT PLAN— July 1988 to December 1988

1. Allergy testing & phenal therapy
2. Oxyidative therapy
3. Interferon and staphage lysate (SPL) injections
4. Vitamin, mineral and amino acid therapy
5. Hormonal therapy

6. Weekly Reiki healing sessions outside the clinic - (my idea)
7. Singing - (my idea)

A description of treatment is in Appendix A.

Phase II Of My Treatment — November to May 1989

As I finally began feeling better, I would drive myself to the clinic, and when I came home I could actually make dinner. This was quite an improvement from the early phase of my treatment. After an informal dinner party, my first cooking effort for friends, I suffered an anaphylactic shock from some kind of insect bite. After being rushed to the hospital over this ordeal, I had a strong intuitive sense that I should discontinue having any more oxygen drips. I didn't know exactly why, but maybe my system had had enough. Both outer circumstances and my own body were giving me a message. Now I would have to find other ways to work with the healing process. One thing I learned again and again through the course of my recovery was that the listening to myself, to my body and my psyche, were as influential to my healing as any rational or intellectual reasoning about a course of action to take next.

When I fully recovered from the bite and the resulting anaphylactic shock, I called the clinic staff and described my harrowing experience. From what I described it was determined that I was developing an allergic reaction to one of the ingredients in the I.V. drip. A later examination proved I had become allergic to the germanium. Because I felt my body becoming intolerant to this procedure, I needed to take a break from it, let my body rebalance, and then assess how I felt.

It is difficult to know when a helpful treatment is enough but I was learning how to monitor myself. No one else can really tell us what to do about our bodies. We have to take the time to know and feel how our body works. It takes a great deal of trial and error, but for anyone with CFIDS or any other immune-related disease it is clearly the one thing we must learn. You will get lots of advice from everyone, especially advice from medical professionals, but you must still rely on the still, quiet voice inside you. A serious allergic reaction, and another near death situation spoke clearly to me.

Discontinuing the I.V. oxidation drips marked a major change in my treatment process. My new treatment plan, lasting about five months, included the following changes:

Phase II Treatment Plan— November to May 1989
1. Acupuncture and auto son treatments
2. Self administered B-12 shots
3. Vitamin, mineral and amino acid therapy
4. Monthly meetings with the doctor
5. Weekly Reiki healing sessions, outside the clinic
6. Progoff journal writing and dream work

A description of treatment is in Appendix B.

Phase III Of My Treatment
In 1989 Dr. Paul Cheney testified before Congress about Chronic Fatigue Syndrome. With Chronic Fatigue Immune Dysfunction Syndrome, he said, an abrupt loss of health and vitality in a previously healthy adult, a prolonged course without clear-cut resolution, and the unusual loss of cognitive skills is seen almost without exception in what is termed the "classic case."

While there is no single test which is always abnormal in patients with CFIDS and always normal in healthy controls, there are patterns of abnormalities seen primarily in the immune system and in the central nervous system. Im-

mune system dysfunction could account for every symptom seen in CFIDS, including those of central nervous system origin.[1]

When I read Dr. Cheney's testimony before Congress, I was impressed by his emphasis on the disease attacking the central nervous system. This would account for all the psychological problems and depression I had experienced. Other research indicated that the disease produced lesions on the brain. These abnormal areas in the brain would disrupt normal brain functioning and would account for my erratic, emotional behavior. I decided after reading this information that I needed to talk more to my doctor about the effect of the disease on my brain and on my psychological behavior, and about my general progress.

In May 1989, I arrived at the clinic with the usual set of questions about my progress, but this time my primary question was, "Why was I not sustaining my energy level all day long?" I could work for only a half a day. I generally had enough energy to do things in the morning, but by noon my energy would drop and I would have to sleep for the rest of the day. I was basically functionless in the afternoons. I became frustrated because as I started getting more energy, I would do more, and then I would have to go to bed for a day or two. My life lacked a balanced flow and a productive rhythm. Projects I started were left incomplete. My desk was covered with stacks of unsorted and unfiled paper. I was always canceling engagements at the last moment. I disliked being inconsistent and not getting things done.

The doctor was also concerned with my inconsistent energy level; he couldn't figure out why I didn't have more stamina. He had rerun all the tests and found that my Epstein-Barr titers were close to the normal range: my anemia report came back good: my thyroid T3 and T4 indicators were within the normal range: and, my estrogen and progesterone levels were fine. My major body complaint was that I had a sore lower back in the area of the kidneys, and I had difficulty sleeping because of this. The chiropractor at the clinic said the soreness wasn't from any structural problem.

The doctor suggested that I take another test, one that he had recently started giving to his CFIDS Patients — the ACTH urine test for the adrenal glands. As he explained the test I knew he was onto something. Stress plays an integral part in CFIDS, and the adrenal glands are the primary agents when the body is called upon to respond to stress. I also knew that the adrenals sit on top of the kidneys and this was the area of soreness.

The adrenals are recognized as one of the body's most important endocrine glands. These glands produce hormonal substances that go directly into the bloodstream. The adrenal glands are composed of two parts, the medulla (inner portion) and the cortex (outer surrounding portion). The medulla and cortex produce many substances, the most important of which are epinephrine, produced by the medulla, and the hormones produced by the cortex. The cortex produces the hormones cortisone and aldosterone. Stress on the body stimulates the adrenal medulla to increase epinephrine production. This hormone increases the secretion of adrenocorticotropic hormone (ACTH) by the pituitary gland, which in turn activates the adrenal cortex to produce cortisone. The function of cortisone in our system is to regulate the metabolism of fats, carbohydrates, sodium, potassium, and proteins. The doctor repeated that without a sufficient supply of cortisone the body dies. After the appointment as I re-listened to the audio tape from our session I realized that if I didn't have enough cortisone I wasn't metabolizing the foods I was taking in, and therefore wasn't getting the energy I needed to sustain me though out the day. I also recognized that if my adrenal glands were not functioning properly, my resistance to stress and resuming a productive life could not happen. Needless to say I was very eager to get the results of this test.

During the two month I waited for the test results, we traveled to our daughter's wedding in Seattle. This was the first time I had been on an airplane in two years. I had difficulty dealing with crowds in the airport and, at the wedding, and I had to leave the reception because I couldn't handle the noise, the live band, the dancing and all the excited energy of people. I was exhausted.

After returning home, I began to lose weight very rapidly. I looked at my eating patterns, but couldn't account for the weight loss except that I eliminated sugar and bread from my daily diet. My skin was beginning to sag noticeably on my face and arms. When I went into a dress shop to try on some clothes I found out that I was down two dress sizes.

The test results finally came back; they indicated that I had Addison's disease. I was confused, frightened, and uncertain about this disease meant. The doctor tried to soften the blow by saying that President Kennedy also had had Addison's disease, and that it was an adrenal insufficiency.

I was tested for twelve hormones; the results showed that I was producing only three of them. The doctor informed me that Addison's disease was a physical atrophy or destruction of the adrenal glands themselves. It is a relatively rare disease, and he said that it is difficult to diagnosis because standard medical texts state that clinically Addison's disease does not usually occur unless at least 90% of the adrenal cortex has been destroyed by idiopathic atrophy, granulomatous destruction, or some other destructive process.

The doctor described the medical nature of Addison's disease and how the ACTH test evaluates whether a patient has a significant rise in serum cortisols following the ACTH (a hormone manufactured in the pituitary gland) injection that I had been given during the test. If one has Addison's disease there is minimal or no response from the adrenal glands due to this injection of ACTH.

I then asked the doctor what caused Addison's disease; he replied that 80% of the cases result from autoimmune problems, 20% from tuberculosis, and 3% from stress problems such as reproduction, coloric, psychic, and aerobic stress.

Actually, the doctor sternly recommended that I move to the top of a mountain, away from people, cars, and problems of the world, because I would never be able to handle stress again in my life. I was stunned. In a weak voice I replied that I already lived out in the country away from crowds and big city stress. He said I had worked very hard on getting the CFIDS in line, but that now I needed to concentrate on the adrenal glands. He recommended that I take the hormone I wasn't producing, hydrocortisone. I was shocked, however, that he would recommend taking a synthetic preparation of the hormone. He assured me that since I wasn't manufacturing the hormones, I would not get any negative results, only positive ones. I was concerned about getting the moon face and other side symptoms of taking cortisone. There had been publicity about athletes using hydrocortisone and about the destructive effects of it on their bodies. I found out later that athletes do not take cortisol steroids.

With the test results indicating I had Addison's disease, I felt like another brick had landed on me. This time the brick was a life-threatening disease. I began to do my own research on Addison's disease and found some strong connections to the pattern of autoimmune diseases that many are getting. This disease is found in people at any age, and affects both sexes with equal frequency. However, the condition that I had, the atrophy of the adrenal glands, came directly from an autoimmune mechanism.

As I studied the medical data about Addison's disease, I found that when a person has this condition they have circulating in their blood adrenal antibodies, thyroid antibodies, parathyroid, and/or gonadial tissue. These circulating antibodies have the direct effect of destroying T-lymphocytes, these important white blood cells that are part of the immune system. These T-lymphocyte cells mount specific types of defenses against invading organisms or viruses that penetrate the body's general defense systems against disease. With Addison's disease the T-lymphocyte part of the immune system is progressively destroyed so that one is unable to resist all types of diseases and viruses.

As I explored more of the implications of Addison's disease, I came to believe that the presence of the condition may be one of the unknown reasons why some people don't get better even after undergoing many of the same positive treatments that I had been given at the clinic.

The Effects of Addison's Disease

To understand Addison's disease is to first understand the hormonal interaction. The hypothalamus gland has nerve cells that manufacture hormones called paraventricular CHR. These hormones communicate to the pituitary gland and carry hormone messages that stimulate the pituitary to make another hormone, ACTH. ACTH is then sent to the adrenal glands where three steroid hormones are then manufactured. The first one is to help the kidneys retain salt so that we are able to live outside the sea. The second is the male sex hormone, and the third is cortisone, a hormone that everyone needs because of its regulatory action in the metabolism of fats, carbohydrates, sodium, potassium, and proteins.

In Addison's disease, because of a lack of hydrocortisone, large amounts of ACTH and CRH are produced. When ACTH increases we may have hyperpigmentation (where the skin changes radically all over the body), and when the CRH increases it may account for depression, which I experienced. The lack of hydrocortisone also produces digestive problems, low physical energy, inability to handle stress, and various types of psychological problems.

In Addison's disease there is also an increased incidence of chronic lymphocytic thyroiditis, or Hashimoto's disease. I definitely had Hashimoto's thyroiditis as indicated from earlier tests. The prognosis in Addison's disease is that it is life-threatening. First, there is destruction of the adrenal glands, next, hyperpigmentation, and, lastly, cachexia (malnutrition), coma, and death. In 1945 hydrocortisone was discovered and eliminated the deaths of Addison's disease patients. But I also learned some important facts. First, taking hydrocortisone over a prolonged period of time and in high dosages, can cause diabetes mellitus, glaucoma, osteoporosis, peptic ulcer, fluid retention, weight gain, acne, muscle weakness, and mood changes. After sorting through all this information it took me a full month to decide whether or not to take the hydrocortisone. Everything I read said that I should take a hormone replacement. I decided to try it and went back to the doctor to get a prescription. I must have made the right decision because a year later, when I was well on my way to full recovery, David told me that the doctor had told him that if I hadn't made the decision to take it I would have died within two months.

Upon taking the hydrocortisone I immediately began to feel better. My energy and physical stamina would now last through the whole day. Of particular relief to both David and me was the diminishing of my emotional swings and the overwhelming depression that I had experienced for such a long time. The discovery of my Addison's disease and the rebuilding of my adrenals with hydrocortisone opened a new chapter in my healing and recovery. I moved forward regaining a normal life after an ordeal of nearly three years.

Phase III Treatment Plan: August 1989 to May 1990

1. Hydrocortisone, and DHEAS
2. Massage
3. Colonics
4. Herbalism
5. Candida diet (2 months)
6. Music — piano and singing
7. Creating a research project
8. Exercise
9. Journal writing

A description of treatment is in Appendix C.

Update — CFIDS Research

In 1990 The First International Conference on Chronic Fatigue Syndrome and Fibromyalgia was held in Los Angeles, California. Dr. Ronald Herberman, Professor at the Cancer Institute of the University of Pittsburgh, described an outbreak of CFIDS in a symphony orchestra. Herberman reported that not only did CFIDS patients display lowered natural killer cell activity but so did healthy spouses and co-workers. The implication was that an infectious agent may be responsible for causing the syndrome. He also reported that this group of relatively young and healthy individuals developed cancers at a rate that was 27 times higher than would be expected for this group.

On May 14, 1990 Time magazine published "Stalking a Shadowy Assailant," by Linda Williams. In this article on chronic fatigue Williams wrote, *"The symptoms are bad enough: sluggishness, sore muscles, fever, headaches, and depression, but on top of that people who suffer from chronic fatigue syndrome often have to endure accusations of hypochondria."*[2] Williams pointed out that the U.S. Government was finally starting to take CFIDS seriously.

In a study published in the April 1991 issue of the *Proceedings of the National Academy of Sciences,* a team of researchers, including scientists at the Wistar Institute headed by Elaine DeFreitas, Paul Cheney, and David Bell, reported their research on CFIDS at the 11th International Congress of Neuropathology in Kyoto, Japan. They discovered evidence of a retrovirus in more than 75% of 31 CFIDS patients studied. In their research CFS patients had blood cells containing a viral sequence similar to the HTLV-II virus. This virus is a retrovirus which is in the same family of viruses that includes the HIV believed by most scientists to cause AIDS, rare types of leukemia and other blood cancers.

In November, 1991 there was a teleconference presenting a variety of researchers and physicians investigating

CFIDS. These researchers discussed the epidemiology, etiology, and treatment of CFIDS and provided the latest research developments. The teleconference was sponsored by over 40 CFID support groups in different locations around the United States. In addition to presenting current information, the teleconference permitted an exchange of questions and opinions by the participants. It was both encouraging and empowering for those of us CFIDS patients who have been both victims and objects of ridicule by the medical community to finally be in dialogue with them.

It was clear from this conference, and from the growing reports and stories in the media about the syndrome, that chronic fatigue is no longer considered a yuppie flu. And, at a very practical level, statistics show that chronic fatigue is not just an upper middle class, white, professional women's disease. The studies show that all socioeconomic levels are being affected by this disease. **At this time the medical community states there is no definitive test for the disease, no agreed upon prevention, and no cure. In 1991, it is still unknown how widespread the disease is throughout the population.** From statistics being reported by the National Disease Center in Atlanta, Georgia, however, CFIDS is five times more prevalent than AIDS, 10 times more prevalent than Alzheimer's disease, and 30 times more prevalent than multiple sclerosis. What we know is that AIDS can be prevented and multiple sclerosis can be diagnosed. Part of the confusion about CFIDS is that it goes by many different names, such as:

    Chronic infectious mononucleosis
    Chronic Epstein-Barr syndrome
    Royal free disease
    Icelandic disease
    Epidemic neuromyasthenia

Post viral (fatigue) syndrome
Limbic encephalopathy
Myalgic encephalomysasthenia

Retrovirus

One of the most significant pieces of research appeared about CFIDS in the spring of 1991. Dr. Elaine DeFreitas from the Wistar Institute, who reported this discovery, indicated that in her research 75% of CFIDS cases showed evidence of a retrovirus in their nervous systems that was related to the retrovirus HTL VII, and was actively being replicated within the DNA of the patient. She and her research team discovered the retrovirus in the peripheral blood and in the sequences in the DNA. They found that the retrovirus was actively expressing itself in a viral sequence pattern commonly associated with retrovirus behavior.

This is the first time that an ubiquitous, viral agent has been associated with chronic fatigue. Generally, a retrovirus is in a small portion of the population and is not casually transmitted from person to person. This research is indicating that this retrovirus, like AIDS, is moving through the general population. The hallmark of this disease is that it creates significant immunological abnormalities and breaks down immune defenses.

Retroviruses are first found in the central nervous system before they are found in the blood. Because of this they are neurotropic in that they influence the nervous impulses of an organ or body structure, creating a variety of neurological problems. The neuroendocrine system responds to the stress of these retroviruses by triggering other infectious viruses which have been latent in the patient's system. With the immune system impaired by the retrovirus, there is little defense to prevent these other viruses from creating a variety of infections and organ malfunctions. The Lancet research article of September 1991 says, *"Unless the immune system is brought back into balance, however, this chronic activation affects the individual further and might eventually lead to other clinical illnesses."*[3]

One example of how the retrovirus puts stress on a system is with the hypothalamus. When under stress by the retrovirus, the hypothalamus is over-stimulated and the hormone CRH is secreted in excess, thereby creating depression. It also doubles the cortisone secreted by the adrenals, creating anxiety; some 60% of the CFIDS patients in the study had psychiatric disorders. Because of the retrovirus affecting the nervous system and the brain directly, these mental disorders are seen as a major component of the disease.

We know that the brain and the immune system communicate directly with each other. An immune cell has a receptor in the cell that is connected to a neuropeptide on the cell wall. These immune system cells are spread throughout the body with their cell walls in constant contact with the cell walls of other tissue and organs. We find these specific immune cells in the tonsils, adenoids, thymus gland, lymph nodes, bone marrow, the white blood cells (monocytes, lymphocytes B-cells, T-cells), other cells of the lymphatic circulation system, the spleen, the appendix, and patches of lymphoid tissue in the intestinal tract. In a sense the immune cells, as they are spread throughout the body, are constantly eavesdropping on a person's inner dialogue — thoughts, feelings, and emotions. The immune cells then respond to the physical as well as to the psychological changes that go on within us. In some sense these receptor cells become the communication link to the psyche.

Again, from a medical research point of view, we begin to regain through this understanding of immune cell intelligence the basic body/mind interrelationship that must be understood for significant healing to take place. Much of what I learned through the psychological and spiritual journey I took to heal and recover from CFIDS, I believe was communicated to my body, to these receptors in the immune cells that "heard" that I was both earnest and serious about getting to the deeper causes in my soul that were creating the physical illness I was experiencing.

PART IV

THE JOURNEY INTO MYSELF

*The body reflects the attitudes of the mind.
Improve the function of the body and you must
improve the state of mind....*
                                    Moshe Feldenkrais

At the same time I worked to get my body healthy, I was
also trying to understand the meaning of my illness.
Journal writing on the days I could write and recording my
dreams helped clarify and bring insights to these feelings.
I found my dreams seemed to follow my emotional life and
also brought clarity out of what was bothering and upset-
ting me on some deeper level of my consciousness.

As my physical condition improved, I was able to read
again. Two books were recommended during the early
stages of my illness. Marion Woodman's *Addiction To
Perfection* offered the first clarification about the process
I had been going through, beyond merely experiencing a
debilitating illness. One of the passages from her book that
gave me direction and hope read: *"A living creature obeys
its own inner laws, moves through cycles of growth, dies
and is reborn as a new creature. We plant our bulbs, water
them and watch them grow. We marvel at them coming
from under the snow. Why should we have more faith in the
bulb than in ourselves."*[1]

From reading Woodman I began to realize that I was
going through some sort of death and rebirth process as I
struggled with the illness. I begin to realize that maybe I
wasn't dying physically, but rather that some inner process was changing inside of me. I kept asking, "How is this
inner change coming about within me?" While I was in this

mood of questioning, the second book came to me, *Descent to the Goddess: A Way of Initiation for Women* by Sylvia Brinton Perera. In the book Perera describes seven steps one takes down inside to find the "goddess." The descent down to my near death with CFIDS felt like I had, as well, taken similar steps.

Perera tells the story of the Goddess Inanna, Queen of the Great Above, and, her sister, Erashkigal, Queen of the Underworld. Erashkigal's world was known as the land of no return. When Inanna heard that her sister's husband had died, she wanted to go to the funeral. But her sister, Erashkigal, told the gate keeper to the Underworld to treat her sister like any other person going through the gates. The book is a description of how all of Inanna's being is stripped away as she goes through each of the seven gates down into the Underworld.

Perera uses an ancient Sumerian poem about Inanna and Ereshkigal to look at the dismemberment that occurs when a woman sheds her identification, dies to an old way of being, and waits for rebirth. First, Inanna must travel through mud that pulls the gold from her ears, then through granite arms that rip the shirt from her breast. Further down into the Underworld, fire singes the hair from her head as she then goes through iron that takes off her limbs. Farther down still, Inanna is thrown into emptiness that sucks her blood. At last she stands in front of Ereshkigal's unpitying eye which freezes her heart and pulls the flesh from her bones as she falls into the Abyss.

As I reflected on the seven gates in Perera's book, I recognized that I had entered into a similar process of having much of my being striped away. I got insights about my death process by sitting for many hours in the silence, and from images that surfaced during my Reiki healing sessions. I would then draw what I had seen or felt, and also write about them in my journal. In the days following I would think about how these ideas applied to my life.

I began to see how my physical body, my mind, and the spiritual, or sacred, aspects of myself were connected in a strange and magical synchronistic process. This interrelated awareness was magnified as I reread sections of my journal and dream writings. I began to see that there were connecting patterns between my illness and deeper issues that I had been avoiding all my life. I was both frightened and exhilarated by this. As these patterns emerged from my reflection and daily struggle with CFIDS, thoughts surfaced that perhaps I really was a part of some grand scheme, or achetypical pattern that both I, and everyone else was connected to. As I worked more with my inner world, I understood that what I was encountering was not so different from the archetypical patterns of the Goddesses that Perera had described.

Reviewing writings from my daily journal and dream log, I discovered my own seven step progression through the gates of the Underworld. I created a description of my own journey into the depths of my being, naming my process the *Seven States of Death*. I believe that this process into and out of death is part of the inner healing of immune and autoimmune diseases. I am convinced that our outer, biological, problems reflect our inner, psychological, problems since we know the cells of the immune system are overhearing the talk by the brain/mind and visa versa. The physical body mirrors our thoughts. For us to heal our physical illness we need to heal the deep roots of our psyche.

Just as I worked with great effort and discipline to understand and heal my physical body, I had to apply the same dedication to the psychological and spiritual aspects of myself. This was very difficult. I wanted to give up on both tasks but, in some strange way, the little steps of healing on one side brought growth and healing to the other side. Actually, for those of us with immune diseases, working on the spiritual and psychological side of our lives may be the most critical part of the healing process. This becomes paramount because many of the reasons for getting the physical illness are directly related to the impoverished condition of our inner life. The more we — as women in particular — learn to go through these *Seven States of Death,* the more we can help heal both ourselves and our impoverished, ailing planet.

THE SEVEN STATES OF DEATH

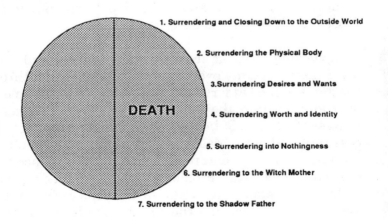

1. Surrendering and Closing Down to the Outside World
2. Surrendering the Physical Body
3. Surrendering Desires and Wants
4. Surrendering Worth and Identity
5. Surrendering into Nothingness
6. Surrendering to the Witch Mother
7. Surrendering to the Shadow Father

THE SEVEN STATES OF DEATH
   1. Surrendering and Closing Down to the Outside World
   2. Surrendering the Physical Body

3. Surrendering Desires and Wants
4. Surrendering Worth and Identity
5. Surrendering into Nothingness
6. Surrendering to the Witch Mother
7. Surrendering to the Shadow Father

1. Surrendering And Closing Down The Outside World

As I look back now, I can trace the closing down of the outer world around me because it eventually made such a strong impact on my psyche. At first, the pulling back process was slow and subtle. I hardly noticed the choices I made that separated me from the outside world. For example, in my counseling work I remember being bored and wishing my clients would talk less. I was getting discouraged and impatient at their slowness, and at their unwillingness to act on what we had been talking about for months. I was losing interest in their stories, and I seemed to be play-acting the therapy situation, rather than being honestly concerned and involved in the process with them. I then began to feel guilty. Both my heart and enthusiasm were gone for listening to people's problems all day.

What was true in my counseling practice was even more pronounced with the work I did in the corporate world. My husband, David, and I sometimes worked together giving workshops with business clients. I would get bored and sleepy, particularly in the afternoons. I could hardly stay awake, and I felt embarrassed about my behavior. Repeatedly, I would ask David to take over my presentations and facilitate the group. I had no idea at this time, however, that I had a physical problem, but, gradually the fatigue of the disease was overtaking me. I fantasized that I would stop working, go off in the woods somewhere by myself, and just meditate. At the time I was unable to clearly interpret these signs of boredom with my counseling clients, the tiredness of working with business clients, or even the fantasy that I wanted to escape from both. I mostly ignored these feelings and body sensations, not really being aware of them, until the signals intensified. I wasn't paying attention to the message my body was trying to tell me.

The boredom, loss of interest, difficulty concentrating, thoughts of being in the country or at the seashore grew stronger and more insistent. I was easily irritated and became more impatient with people, and or situations. I would wake up feeling depressed, and I wondered why. Now, I know that these feelings and behaviors were a clear signal that my inside world needed attention. My heart was telling me to close down to the outside world for awhile in order to make room for something new to enter. Intellectually I had heard or read about the notion of listening to yourself, and indeed, I had meditated for years in order to be more aware and conscious. But, because of the gradual way in which the physical and emotional signals began to emerge I was unable to recognize them as they were happening to me.

I once heard a story of a therapist whose practice was slowing down. His clients were spontaneously leaving him without any real reason. One night he awoke and heard a voice saying, "You must let go of these clients in order to let the new ones come who need to see you." Some inner voice was also telling me to let go, but I was having difficulty hearing it. The slow, almost imperceptible breakdown of that which has given us meaning and fulfillment in our lives is the doorway through which we enter this first condition or state of death. This is the beginning of the surrendering process, or the dying to our old forms and patterns of experience. I believe that we often think that it is someone or something else that is making the change in our life. "If I had more time off, or if I had a different partner, or if I could change jobs, or if I had more money, or if, or if, or if . . ." We don't want to believe, or at least we aren't conscious of recognizing that we are responsible for causing our world to crumble. I think this process of going inward is initiated from a deeper, clearer, but unconscious part of our self. It is this part of us that knows what our next step is, and knows what is best for us.

Once David and I moved away from the city to the country, the closing down process was blatant. It was not a subtle experience for me anymore. We lived eight miles from the nearest town, on a winding country road. Our neighbors were far removed. We were in a dry foothills environment; I was used to moist green trees of the coast with lots of birds singing in them. The weather was hot and dry, and, of course, I hated hot and dry weather. Physically, I do much better in cool, moist environments. I was experiencing an environment that was against my nature. It was foreign country, definitely not familiar territory that offered comfort and inner support.

When we first arrived and settled into our new home, the quietness of the country was deafening. There wasn't a bird's song, or even a bird in sight! There was little wind movement, other than an occasional breeze. Our home was on a lake with fish in it, but even the lake seemed lifeless. Looking back on that time, I believe that the lifelessness I saw around me was a reflection of the growing inner deadening of my psyche. My familiar outside world began to collapse rapidly from what I had known before. I had no friends here and it was difficult to work because this necessitated a nearly four hour commute. Added to this traumatic environmental change was the difficulty selling my house in the Bay Area. As I dragged my emotional feet in selling the house, all kinds of unimaginable problems emerged.

The stress on my body increased as I resisted and struggled against breaking away from my old ways of living, and in losing my identity as a professional, frontier's woman. I got scared as I finally began to become aware that the wonderful world I knew had been destroyed — it was gone. The loneliness of being away from a familiar cosmopolitan life, far from cherished friends, far from weather that I liked, and far from my comfortable, refined lifestyle ultimately wore me down. But even with my deep weariness, I struggled against letting go and surrendering — I didn't want to be put away into a quiet, country monastery.

Later, after this period of collapse and rebellion, I came across St. John's book, *The Dark Night of the Soul.* In one of the passages he speaks to this place of collapse of one's outer world in which I had arrived, both through the move to the country and the emergence of my illness. St. John suggests,

> *If souls to whom this comes to pass know how to be quiet at this time and trouble not about performing any kind of action whether inward or outward, neither have any anxiety about doing anything, then they would delicately experience this inward refreshment that ordinarily, if a man have desire or care to experience it he experiences it not. It does its work when the soul is most at ease and freest from care. It is like the air if one would close one's hand upon it, escapes.*[1]

I was being forced to go into quietness. It would take me a long while, however, before I could have any "ease" with it, as St. John suggests. I had entered into a spiritual dying process that has a long tradition and is described in many spiritual teachings throughout the world. I didn't know this cutting off of the outer world had meaning and purpose to it. I was frightened and alone inside a cage that I didn't want to be in. I had no guidelines as how to work with these strange new conditions in my life, and I had no sense of what was going to happen. Because I was not listening, as with Inanna, Queen of the Great Above, the gold was being stripped from my ears.

2. Surrendering The Physical Body

One year before we moved to the country, I first noticed pain and stiffness in my right hip and groin. This eventually got so bad that I went to an acupuncturist, a chiropractor, my medical internist, and then to all kinds of unusual practitioners. I even had two psychic healers attempt to perform healings on me. I was determined to heal this condition, but nothing seemed to help. Because of this problem, I had difficulty doing aerobics, yoga, and swimming. I eventually went to a physical therapist to treat my hip condition. The physical therapist was surprised at how limber I was. I sensed that she thought I was a hypochondriac, and without saying so directly, implied that there was really nothing wrong with me.

When we moved to the high country the pain in my arms, and especially my shoulder joints, intensified. The acupuncturist had said that it was not unusual for older women to have shoulder joint problems. He said it was an accumulation of calcium in the joints. So, I thought the pain was just the result of getting older, and that I needed to exercise with weights so the calcium wouldn't accumulate. But the more I tried to exercise the worse the pain got; rather than feeling invigorated, I felt tired and even exhausted at times.

I found myself being forced to surrender to the physical body's deep felt tiredness. I fought it, and denied that I was really tired. But I had become so chronically tired that I didn't feel rested even after a long night's sleep. Then, there were also the many nights waking up in terror and sweating. I would wake up exhausted and all I wanted to do was sleep.

Surrendering to the many symptoms of the illness came next. The flu symptoms appeared first, followed by indigestion, then by a tightness in my throat that continually made me feel like I was about to hyperventilate. As the physical symptoms accumulated, other fears began to surface. I began to fear the occurrence of a periodic vibration in my chest — I thought I was going to have a heart attack. There were broader fears about being unable to function at work and at home any longer. There were fears about losing my mental capacities, about feeling old, and as I looked into the mirror, the fact that I was looking old. I was fearful that my body would never be normal again because of my sore, stiff arms and the difficulty this created when I dressed. The stiffness was also causing me to struggle to get in and out of the car, and I had great difficultly walking to the top of the stairs in the house.

It actually took an entire 12 months of body suffering and emotional denial before I could allow myself to accept the fact that I was physically ill, and that I possibly would never get better or have a normal life again. I was utterly devastated. I hated my body. I felt victimized by my body as I confronted my mortality for the first time. Slowly, I began to accept the fact that I couldn't change my body by being angry at it. At some point I surrendered to the reality: I had to live with my physical condition a day at a time. Once I stopped denying and fighting it, and, after I surrendered to being ill without anger or self pity, help came to me to begin the healing process.

I remember feeling pretty good one day, so I decided to ride my bicycle. As I started out I felt great. I had energy and stamina, and I pedaled up and down the first hills easily. After a few more hills I began to tire: but I was determined to finish my ride. I pushed forward and rode around to the other side of the lake. I did it! But then it was all I could do to make it back to the house. From the far side of the lake I had to walk the bike. My energy was totally gone, but I had to somehow make it back home. I literally had to crawl up the stairs of the house. Sobbing and barely able to move, I felt emotionally drained and very ill. When David found me he couldn't believe what had happened. For several days all I could do was lie down and do nothing. I had no idea at that time that the more one exercises the more the virus is active and multiplies. My body must have been flooded with viruses from the exertion. I felt like I was dying. The surrender to the body, was saying, "Yes I was sick, I was unable to do what I had done before and maybe would never do them again, this was difficult to admit and accept."

On looking back at this period, my body was asking for a moderation of physical activities. My body was asking me not to do as much as I had been used to doing. This was a request for a different use of my energy. I needed to be more selective in the way I pushed and used my energy. Now, I use my energy to bring things to me rather than pushing so hard to get them to happen. I now ask internally for another force to work on my behalf, and the same things come to me with much less effort. Also, I don't let myself get to extreme low points. As I feel myself begin to get low emotionally or physically, I stop what I am doing and change course. I let my body do what it wants to do, instead of pushing it so hard with my mind and my will.

I had never paid much attention to the rhythms of my body. I didn't have a clear sense of what was going on with it. My attention had always been on the outside world. I thought that somehow the body just took care of itself. I didn't realized that the foundation to everything in life was a sound body. How did I lose this attention to my body? How did I lose the ability to hear the sensations and the messages my body was giving me?

I began to understand that part of the problem is the cultural and societal training we go through, as women, to focus only on our outer image. We are apparently supposed to maintain our female image by using makeup, styling our hair, keeping slim, having face lifts, breast implants, doing our fingernails, and wearing beautiful clothes. Knowing whether the body is really hungry, analyzing what it wants to eat, or, what is the reason for the headache, backache, and heartache is not encouraged in our society. We are encouraged to take an aspirin and block the symptoms rather than encouraged to learn how to listen to our bodies. By learning to listen to my body, however, I am now able to know which side of my head the pain is on, and what may be the actual cause of the headache. The headache may mean my colon is disturbed, or that it is my ovulation time, or that I am being affected by a certain type of stress.

All my life I have expended lots of energy toward other people; I would give my all to everyone. During my three year bout with CFIDS, I learned how to monitor my energy level, a concept introduced to my by a music conductor. He described how to anticipate a big crescendo at the end of a musical piece. At rehearsal, the conductor would explain, "Don't give all of your voice and breath as you sing. Save the energy of your voice and breath during the piece even though it calls for a certain level of exertion. Save the energy for the end crescendo where you want to give full impact of the piece to the audience." He was teaching us both moderation and selectivity.

I believe the reason I gave my all to everyone was so that

I would be liked and be seen as "wonderful" in their eyes. I also know that doing things for approval made me feel good. I was addicted to approval for the good feeling, just as an alcoholic is addicted to drinking alcohol.

Gloria Steinem suggests that we are in the third decade of the second wave of feminism. The first wave was to establish legal identity and the second wave is to unblock the barrier to a woman's inner garden. In her work *Revolution from Within: A Book of Self Esteem*, Steinem writes,

> *Socialization determines the way this self-hatred is played out: females tend to grow up to mistreat themselves; males tend to grow up to mistreat others. . . Educating girls more like boys—that is, to express anger and stand up for themselves instead of turning it into self injury and depression—would diminish self-punishment.*[1]

Just as with Inanna in Sylvia Brinton Perera's recounting of the descent to the Underworld, the shirt was being ripped from my breast.

3. Surrendering Wants And Desires

Surrendering to the current condition of my physical body led me next into the areas of my impulses, my addictions, and my self discipline. I very quickly began to discover, because of the results of the medical tests, that many of the things I had accepted as natural I could do no longer. I suddenly uncovered a hidden bag of wants and desires, and if I kept trying to fulfill these desires, I would not regain optimum health. Here ensued a deep, inner emotional battle to give up things I really liked and that gave me a great deal of pleasure. I learned, however, that many of these pleasures were not only killing me, they were salves to emotional hurts and wounds locked deep within my psyche.

The first set of desires that I had to confront was my eating patterns. First, I had an insatiable sweet tooth. I loved ice cream, chocolate, cakes, and desserts of all kinds. Yes, I felt good when I ate sweets. When I felt down or depressed, I ate something sweet as a pick-me-up. Since I had never experienced a serious weight problem, I never thought anything about my sugar habit until, several years earlier when I was diagnosed as having hypoglycemia. But I believed I was keeping it under control. I was devastated, though, when I went to the Preventive Health Clinic in 1988 and learned from the allergy testing that I was allergic to the 24 foods that I enjoyed the most. The mandate to no longer eat these foods was like taking away my favorite toys. It wasn't until I was forced by my illness to stop eating these particular foods that I begin to understand how addicted I really was. Sugar was in everything I loved. I was a sugar addict. And, like any addict, I suffered the emotional withdrawals. And like anyone on a twelve step program, I still take it a day at a time.

This allergic reaction is an autoimmune problem. When the immune system isn't functioning properly it reacts in an exaggerated manner to different things. The immune system's basic purpose is to form antibodies against harmful substances. Our allergic or sensitive reactions to certain foods results from the immune system attacking the chemicals from these foods that are producing harm to our system. We can get sensitive to the foods we repeatedly eat because our immune system thinks the food's chemical base is antigens (foreign substances) that are attacking us. As the immune system constantly overreacts to a continual stimulation of the same kind of food, it loses its protective ability to resist the harmful chemicals in these foods. It is then unable to continue to maintain good health in our bodies. The continuous chemical from the food, like sugar, overwhelms the antigens so that there is no resistance to the sugar in the system. Other viral and bacterial agents can then more easily invade and make us sick. This high use of sugar in our diet is part of why I believe we constantly get colds, flus and every other kind of contagion that is continually moving through the population.

In the case of *"auto"* immune disease a person must attack themselves. I was attacking myself by continuing to eat a diet of sugar-filled foods which I was allergic to. My immune system then, was over worked trying to protect me. We also have a type of emotional immune system that protects us against abuse, rejection, and loneliness. This part of my immune system was also not functioning well. My mind began to attack the weaker parts of me for several reason: for not having my regular diet, for my erratic sleep patterns, for my drastic change in life style, for my lack of close friends, and my dwindling professional life. My mind said I deserved to have these things in my life and it began to attack the basic level of my wants and desires.

My reaction to the attacks on both my immune systems revealed their deficiencies and I became overly emotional about not having the foods I liked; I felt like an addict on withdrawal. I was a child crying at every simple change; my life was upside down. I went from being with people to being alone: I went from eating in all types of restaurants to eating at home, or, occasionally, at very selected restaurants. I had worked for 30 years outside the home, now I was home all of the time. And the final insult was in having to avoid eating everything I dearly loved, I had to begin eating everything I hated, like oatmeal and rice.

It was difficult to give in to this stage of surrender. But when I did start accepting that I had to give up many of my desires and wants something wonderful and helpful happened. One day, as I was lying on the treatment table, my chiropractor looked at me and said, "You need to nurture yourself. Do you know how to do that?" "Yes," I answered. He replied, "No, you don't, or you wouldn't be so sick." He then told me to go home and do only things that I wanted to do, and, to avoid thinking that I should do, or had to do, anything. "If the dishes need to be done and you aren't in the mood to wash them, leave them in the sink," he said. He also asked me to imagine a time in my life that brought me great joy; I was to remember this joyful event every time I shifted to a new activity during the day.

He offered two clues as to what surrendering to desire was about. First, not to force myself to do something just because I thought I should. And second, to infuse my mind constantly with feelings of joy and well being. Another, and, perhaps, the most important idea was how to nurture myself in practical, simple, easy ways. I decided to experiment with this intriguing notion. First, I allowed myself to lie in a hammock under the ponderosa pine trees overlooking the lake for two days. I read a book, took naps, and played with my dog and cat. Surrendering to what I inwardly wanted and needed to do, instead of allowing the impulses of addictive desires and wants to compulsively drive me, was an incredible shift in awareness and practical focus for me. This experience of surrendering to inner desires allowed me to explore myself on a level that I had never before touched.

I learned that this double surrendering is an important part of the healing process. When something is being taken away, something else will fill its place. But the fear connected with surrendering is the possibility that nothing will fill the void, the emptiness, the pain. The unknown knowledge of death is the fear that keeps us from moving away from death. From this lesson I learned to change the energy behind my behavior. I realized my resistance to the change of desires created the internal struggle that was making me sick. I needed to give up resisting the vast changes I was undergoing. As Inanna, my hair was being singed from my head.

4. Surrendering Worth And Identity

Taking away what I desired and wanted left me with an overwhelming distinct feeling of losing not only myself and my identity, but also not feeling valued or worthy. My familiar, solid foundation was being dismantled, stone by stone, through the illness. "What else is there but my old character and identity," I thought. "This can't be real, this isn't happening to me. Please God, make this whole thing a dream, take it away."

As I struggled letting go of my desires and wants, I descended into a whole different level of surrender. It was not just letting go of who I was because of what I could no longer eat, or places I couldn't go, or people I could no longer visit with. It began to feel like a fundamental attack on who I was as a person. It had to do with how I thought about myself, and what made me a worthwhile member of the universe. What was I going to do with my life?

The first occurrence in which I noticed my identity and worth slipping away was with what I call the "carpenter incident." While David was commuting to the Bay Area, I was alone in the new country house to manage the major house repairs. The carpenter was a country-type man. He wasn't much of a talker, seemed much more comfortable with "men" talk, and hard drinking. I felt he didn't have a high opinion of women, and looked down on them. It may have created conflict if he knew I was a professional woman. It was also difficult with my illness to concentrate and make clear decisions. So I played the lowly housewife to make sure the job got done.

To lose the foundation and core of my life by moving to the country, and to be forced to re-evaluate and rethink my basic values and desires, I began to be overwhelmed by fear and an increasing sense of panic. I had been so proud to be a professional woman, active in counseling, working jointly with David in workshops, conducting television interviews, and the like. The fear of being unable to support myself financially revealed where I had placed my greatest value, priority and self worth. My self image was that of a woman who could take care of herself and be independent financially. "How could this be happening to me?" I would ask myself in disbelief. I would lie in bed and feel as if I was going to tear apart in a crazy mosaic of mismatched pieces. I was terrified that I would be unable to survive without earning money. I would become one of those dependent women, weak and incapable of doing anything for myself.

I had been encouraged by my parents to go to college and get a good paying job. I learned in the 1960s, after a divorce, that I had to take care of myself. Work and taking care of myself financially were the primary bases of my self worth and self esteem. The reinforcement I got from home and the culture was that it was bad to stay home and be a housewife. So now, most of what I valued and felt was important was coming apart, disintegrating, disappearing. I then began to experience deep shame for no longer having any outer value, worth, or identity in the world. I no longer had a meaningful life work. Now, I viewed myself as just a housewife, and a sick one at that. This stripping away of my identity and self worth opened the door to the next step, and to the most frightening part of the process. As Inanna was stripped of her limbs, I fell farther and farther into the Abyss.

5. Surrendering Into Nothingness
The panic and terror of losing total control of my life,

and, watching it disintegrate was horrifying. Was I the antagonist in a horrible monster film? Although at times it seemed unreal, the mental and emotional pain was more than I could handle. I tried to figure out ingenious ways to escape the pain, the feelings of shame, the overwhelming loss of identity. The more I felt out of control physically as well as emotionally, the more I felt as if **"I"** didn't exist. "I am just nothing, a nobody without a meaningful purpose. I don't know if I have the energy to even stay alive." I would sit and stare out the kitchen window at the horse pasture or from the expanse of windows in the living room at the lake trying to figure out why I was put on this earth. Who am I? Am I just here to vegetate? I would ask myself the age-old questions over and over. I felt I was invisible and I would find myself in many situations where people treated me as if I didn't exist.

I can remember one time after David finished talking on the phone to a business friend, I became hysterical. I screamed at him, "Why wasn't I considered in your business discussion that concerned us both? Don't you think my thoughts count? Am I so sick that I don't have a mind?" I raged, screamed, and cried uncontrollably. I felt powerless and like a child. The feelings of powerlessness and loss of control so engulfed my emotions that, in the days following, I felt I was dying.

These emotional outbursts were horrifying to both of us. I no longer knew how to control myself or my emotions. Some uncontrollable part of me had been set loose and some part of me knew that it was putting our marriage relationship in jeopardy as well. It was also separating me from friends and from my life work, self worth and self image. Feelings of loneliness and despair trickled like icy streams of water into my soul. I was consumed by nothingness.

This fall into the Abyss became a total obsession. During
this time I wrote in my journal:

> *The leaving of my life behind makes me lonely,
> unhappy, but I can't go back to it. Why? Because
> it feels flat and dead. Where would I fit in if I went
> back? Could I keep up the pace I had before?
> Could I go back to the Bay Area and buy a condo,
> go to work everyday, have dinner with friends or
> go out to parties, buy outfits to make me look good
> and slide back into the competition. Whew! That's
> a lot of pressure. The question I ask is: Why am
> I trying to get ahead? I have finally come to
> believe that nobody really cares about anyone
> else unless it is important for their own survival.
> It is amazing to me that at each step of life the
> outside world really doesn't care whether we live
> or die, unless you're a somebody. Then if you die
> they can say they knew you. **Basically we are
> all alone,** but I didn't know this until I went
> away from my friends, from my work, and inher-
> ited a sick body. All the activity, all the events,
> and all the work covers up the awareness that we
> basically are all alone in this life. No one is there
> to help me out. I either do it on my own or I don't
> do it. All the people I thought would help me out
> if I needed it just weren't there. I am mad, angry,
> sad, and depressed. All the expensive clothes, the
> fancy ideas, the hard work, and great people that
> I've known have deserted me. **I am alone.***

In his book, *By the Body of the Earth*, Satprem writes,

> *For there is a moment, a point, where we can
> free ourselves, which is like a dying. We are
> already dead, walled up in a circle and con-
> gealed in a bubble. We must overcome a power,
> an amplified selfhood – our own ruthless enemy.
> Our bubble holds in it our nurturing seeds of
> destruction. The force that keeps us from moving
> on to a vaster life. And there is a point of passage,*

an instant when by harnessing the bubble's accu-
mulated power we can pass through in a flash,
and we cross to the other side, or we will die.... We
embark on the wrong path only to find that it is
part of the right one.[1]

The day after I wrote Satprem's words in my journal, I woke up so frightened I called my spiritual healer, Mary, and told her I was shaky, teary, and that a different kind of fear had surfaced. It was more like terror, and a question of life and death. My spiritual healer said I did have a choice concerning whether I would live or die. I didn't want to hear this message, though, and I rushed on to tell her more of my fear: "I don't want to return the call to my mother because I felt she would tell me what to do." Then, when Mary responded I interrupted her again. "I feel like I have no boundaries; it feels like anyone can overpower me and control me." I was out of breath, my breathing ragged and uneasily. There was a long pause; the silence was overwhelming. Then Mary asked, "What is your inner child doing at this moment?"

In our work together, this spiritual healer had helped me focus on the little girl that was hidden deep inside of me. It had been a revelation to realize that there was this child part of me that had not grown up, and was wanting my help and protection as an adult. As I focused inward to that place where I made contact with my inner child, I pictured a tiny little girl inside of me. She seemed to be huddled down next to something, holding her arms around herself trying to comfort herself. When I told Mary, "She seems to be feeling very sad and lonely" Mary said, "Bring her to your heart and give her comfort and love." I returned to the inner image, I tried to see myself walk to her and kneel down and put my arm around her, but the image kept fading. I had a hard time giving her love and comfort. As I kept trying to reach out to her, I saw my little girl refusing to be loved by me. She seemed to be holding her breath in refusal.

Suddenly, I began to feel that I wasn't really letting her in emotionally, and that was why she was refusing me. My spiritual healer, Mary, said she could see a resistance, like armor, around me so that the healing light couldn't come through to touch my inner child. When she asked what I thought the armor could be, I replied that I believe the armor represented being hard on myself. "My head gets in the way of my heart. I feel good and then my head tells me why I can't feel good. Something always seems to pull me down. I block my own energy. When I am not feeling that good feeling about myself, I want others to give it to me, but even then I often don't let them."

Mary said that it sounded like my little child was being locked away from my heart for comfort and support. Later, I began to realize and understand that feeling this numbing nothingness is like our inner child being locked away from our adult selves. The nothingness is that split, that vast separation that Satprem wrote about, between our inner child and our adult self that pretends to be OK. These feelings of nothingness had been deeply embedded in my psyche for a long, long time. Through a series of rebirthing experiences (a therapeutic process that uses a specific type of breathing pattern to trigger off unconscious memories), I began to surface memories that possibly my parents were disappointed that I wasn't a boy. In fact, as a child I was called Patrick on occasion. I believe that often girl babies are greeted with thoughts of, "Oh darn, it's a girl." I was born the wrong gender. My inner girl child never had a chance to really know and believe that she was valued and OK. And although I tried in some ways to be a boy by pleasing my father, I knew unconsciously that I really couldn't be a boy.

Living unconsciously in this in-between "nothing" place begins to catch up with us as women. I remember reading an article, *"Condolences, It's a Girl"* (Time, Fall 1990), about a Chinese woman who said that having a baby girl had destroyed the family; when her husband found she decided to keep the baby girl he left her. And in India, *"Until a few decades ago, the drowning of infant girls was tolerated in poor rural areas as an economic necessity. A girl was just another mouth to feed, another dowry to pay, a temporary family member who would eventually leave to serve her husband's kin. Girls in India are also looked upon by their parents as burdens."*[2]

I began to remember how mother and dad wanted a boy and not a girl child, and how very painful it was for me to be a girl. To allow these images and thoughts from my childhood to come up and be nakedly unmasked to me was horrifying. My guess is that for most women these kind of thoughts and experiences have been pushed far down into the inner psyche, into the darkest corners of our being until our defense system gets so exhausted the truth can hide no longer. This pushing down of painful thoughts and feelings is probably a major strain on the immune defense system. **I now see that for most of my life I have been, one way or another, unconsciously defending being a girl.**

In order to survive in the real world however, my immune system became over-worked and over-stressed because it had to defend myself against myself. It tried to protect both the inner little girl and the adult women, and rationalize unconsciously the vast gap between. As the ability to defend itself began to fail, I developed symptoms of an auto (self-attacking) immune illness. Chaos, rage, and the overwhelming nothingness were hidden beneath the surface of my day to day life. I was using tremendous energy to keep the lid on myself, every waking hour of the day. It was no wonder, then, that my defense or immune system was wearing out. I remember writing in my journal at this time, *"I must stay out of everyone's life in order to go inside to find my own self."* The self that I thought was me was hiding behind a mask in hopes that no one would find out I was a girl. For all of my adult life I had been a professional woman, and I began to realize that being a sophisticated professional was kind of like being a boy. I could keep my professional mask on instead of feeling the pain of nothingness, of not being a boy.

As I became conscious of the gap between my inner little girl and my adult professional self, I believed that nothingness meant having no one who needed me, no one enjoying my presence, and no one appreciating my value or worth. Alone and sick in the country I was forced to go to that nothing place that was both inside and outside of me. When I finally could resist no longer I allowed myself to feel and surrender to the pain and agony of this state. I became like Inanna, thrown into nothingness with blood and energy sucked out of me. I began to search for the issues that were creating this condition in my life.

6. Surrendering To The Witch Mother

As I let myself drop further into the aloneness and nothingness, I was absolutely terrified. I was also angry because I believed that no one cared about me. I felt deserted, abandoned. I felt flat, dull; there was no sweetness in my life. At this time I was going to a sensitive male acupuncturist. I hoped, by increasing my energy flow through the acupuncture process, he would be able to take away my pain — both the physical and emotional. After the treatment with the needles, however, he only increased my emotional pain when he said, "There is a witchlike woman in you." Offended, angry, and defensive I went away vowing to never return to him again.

At first I was repulsed by his statement. Slowly, in the days that followed, though, as I replayed our conversation, his words began to make sense. He also suggested, "It is your mother who has been trying to dominate, control, and demean you." I was able to own that she likes to overprotect and pull the reins close in on me. I was able to own the truth that she is often judgmental, and that she has a critical edge in her voice that comes across as discounting my ideas and my opinions. This tension does not allow us to really communicate, and understand each other. Over the years, then, I learned to close down after negative interactions. She would frequently tell me the "right" way to do something and it made me feel that my way wasn't good enough. Finally, I didn't fight back, instead I would avoid and run from her with the thought, "I am just not good enough." I believe we played out the roles of the classic dominator mother and the perfect subordinate daughter child.

Years before, when I said I wanted to have an adult relationship with her she replied, "I am your mother." And that was that. So, I tried to break the umbilical cord on my own. I wanted to grow up. I wanted to break this inequality of parent and child that existed between us. In *Toward A New Psychology of Women*, Jean Baker Miller writes: "*It is clear then, that the paramount goal is to end the relationship; that is, **to end the relationship of inequality**. The period of disparity is meant to be temporary. People may continue their association as friends, colleagues, or even competitors, but not as 'superior' and 'lesser.' At least this is the goal.*"

From her mother role, I responded to her like a puppet; I allowed her to make my decisions. I discovered as a child, that if I did not follow her lead, I would then hurt her feelings, and thus experience her anger. I then would feel like a bad little girl. I chose to make her happy so she wouldn't get upset and withdraw her love. Over the years, I learned to stay out of her web of "superior" judgments to protect myself from feeling bad. This is the classic co-dependent struggle. Now, being in my middle years I decided that I had had enough. This co-dependent "service" relationship between mother and daughter wasn't right, it wasn't healthy, and I knew it.

Over the years I had developed a strong intuitive and emotionally sensitive personality type in order to cope with her. She is my opposite, being a strong thinking, left-brained, linear personality. As I thought about the different aspects of our relationship from the past, I remembered that as a little girl when I was sick, I would feel comforted by her. I began to understand that I probably got sick just to get this attention and connection with her, in an non-judgmental way. Was I now trying the same strategy of getting sick as an adult to get attention?

The acupuncturist's comment, "The witch mother is affecting your illness," was a clue that, in order to get healthy, I had to do something about this "witch mother" I had internalized into my adult life. I realized that there was my real mother who I had occasional contact with, and, then, this inner mother that I lived with all the time. In some ways, the inner "witch mother" was the one I was really doing battle with. In some ways, however, I could only deal with one mother by dealing with the other one. I had to confront both my real mother and the internalized mother in order to bring my little girl and adult woman together.

At the time I didn't know, consciously, how important this process was for me, but my body knew. Being held so tightly by a mother is very destructive for a woman. The result is that the daughter remains a girl. And, if she is subordinate to her mother she will likely be subordinate to others, like a husband. My anger was directed at my mother and myself because I didn't want to be a little girl anymore, or, subordinate to anyone else. I wanted to grow up.

I learned how to play the sweet, gooey, pleasing game which is exactly what society expects of women. Although I was hurt and angry about letting go of this emotionally unhealthy little girl pattern, I couldn't yet give myself the permission to mature into my own psyche, and gain my own wisdom as a woman, and formulate a new, healthier mythology. I still wanted to believe that I was not strong enough to really be my own person, break the cord, fly out of the nest. In my journal I wrote: "I think my mother has always seen me as weak physically, weak emotionally, and not having the analytical type of thinking that makes one 'smart' in this society. So her obligation is to keep a close watch on me and take care of me. As I experience the overprotective behavior at my age, it looks like control and possession over me."

I began to see the "witch" issue inside of me as a power play. The game focus was about who I would allow to have power over me. An internal struggle of domination, the power game to make me feel less than myself, unsure of myself, not confident, not an equal, and in some fundamental way different from the person I really knew myself to be. I felt intimidated by the "witch mother." I wanted out.

And where did I do all of the struggling about the "witch mother" power game? I literally took to my bed and curled up in a ball, in the fetus position. I was too tired and too ill to get out of bed even to just sit by the window. I would moan, cry, and pull at my bed clothes and at my body from this witchy feeling of possession. I wished and wished that the feeling would vanish, that I would be whisked away and saved somehow from allowing myself to be controlled by other people: from having to be what someone else wanted me to be.

The last straw in this struggle was the breakdown of the body. Like Inanna, the life juice was being sucked away. Thoughts rambled through me: "Oh what pain will I have of letting go of the body? What will happen? Will I die? Would I die if I let myself be totally taken over? If I survived and stayed in this subordinate little girl role at least I would not be alone." To grow up and become an adult woman is having to know aloneness. Experiencing aloneness is part of the initiation of becoming a woman. And this was the power struggle in me. To remain the little girl or to grow up and be a woman.

"What does it mean to become a woman?" I thought. I had no models. I couldn't think about how to do it at this time. I was too caught up in the anger, helplessness, and frustration of trying to allow my witch mother to let go of me, to allow myself to be set free. At the same time, I thought that I could not let go of her. When one is in the subordinate position, as I was, we want the reason and tools for how to live given to us by that authority. I believed that she, as the controller, was the only one who that could let me go.

I would lie in bed and scream "Let me go!" I remember one night sobbing in bed and crying out to be released from this hold so I could go on either living or to dying. I could increasingly feel the "witch mother" inside of me destroying my confidence, my self esteem, my willingness to make decisions on my own without "her" approval. I didn't want to keep trying to please her, or being good, getting her approval, doing what she wanted, agreeing with her, being the perfect little girl. I couldn't do it anymore, and my stomach just wrenched with dry heaves. It literally made me sick, and I had gut wrenching nausea. I felt torn, stretched, and shredded into mismatched pieces of myself by the inner conflict. I prayed to be released. I pleaded, of myself, "Please, please let me go."

These were dark times. This continued for weeks; I became extremely inward, and I hardly even went outside of the bedroom. During the night, the worse times, the feelings would come back to haunt and terrorize me. I would scream to get rid of them. I am sure that anyone else seeing me in this condition would have labeled me as mentally sick. And, of course, I was "mentally" sick. The disease, the toxins, the poisons were coming from the Abyss to the surface, accompanied by a fever and deliriums. As these hot, turbulent feelings began to finally subside, I remember getting a phone call one morning from my mother. I described it in my journal:

I immediately had the feeling of anxiety in my stomach and solar plexus area when I heard her voice. It's as if the fear tightened up my ability to talk, or speak out. As I listen to her begin to speak an old scene came to mind—I had expressed my emotions and upset my mother. She is crying. I get frightened that she is crying. I feel I am responsible for her, and must close off my feelings in order to protect her. As the scene plays itself out I realize that I continually take on the feeling that I've been a bad girl to make her cry. I realize that this constant closing myself down to protect her is part of why I am sick. As I hear the content of my mother's call she is telling me that she has real concern for me in my illness. She goes on to say that she can't tell me her feelings on the phone very easily, so she would write them to me. She says she will do this because that is her most comfortable way to express herself.

I knew from that phone call that I had broken through the sealed bubble. I had gotten not only her attention, but the attention of my inner "witch mother" as well. On the telephone my mother was honest with me. She couldn't express herself the way I do, but she could do it in her own way. After this conversation my emotional "fever" broke. My torment and anxiety left.

As I now understand it, this break and death with the "witch mother," both externally and internally, is a form of initiation that we, as women, have never been given in our culture. We have no formal rites for women. No one tells us that we need to separate, cut the mother-daughter tie, and become whole, complete persons as a result. This does not mean that we totally reject everything in the mother-daughter relationship. Most of us have rejected our mothers out of anger or in our unconscious anger have remained tied to them. Many times the face of the "witch mother" was the same as my real mother. But I began to see that the "witch mother" was more than my birth mother. That until I cut the tie with the "witch mother" I would remain the image of a little girl inside and never become a woman.

Most of us take on our fathers' values instead and accept intimidation as a way of life. As I reviewed my life, I noticed that I also had allowed others both men and women, to control me through intimidation. I had allowed myself to be jerked around by what I believed others thought of me, by what others said about me, and how they spoke to me. Thus, I learned a way of allowing myself to remain intimidated; I had allowed this script, this game, this mythology to run my life.

How did this intense struggle with my inner and outer mother affect my getting ill and staying so sick? Since I was not the dominant one in the most important and fundamental relationship that had shaped my life, that of mother and daughter, I began to play a reverse game of control. I did this by trying to make those who dominated me feel as bad as I did about my being dominated by them. For example, with my husband, David, I would make him feel bad for abandoning me for going to work. I would try to make him feel guilty that he wasn't constantly with me to help me in my sickness. I added a tremendous amount of stress on him by trying to make him feel responsible for my illness. I was into a blaming mode, another game of fear.

I would blame others for my illness, trying to make them feel bad so that I would get the attention I thought I needed. I was playing out a passive aggressive scenario towards others. Deep inside I was angry at them, but outwardly I appeared nice to get them to feel sorry for me. I found that I was usually angry at people who were impersonal, cold, and low in feeling. This was the angry view I projected onto my mother. As I stopped the blaming and projecting game on my mother, on David and on friends, I then began to accept that I alone had to be responsible for the choice of healing myself. By beginning the process of healing the wounds deep inside of my psyche, this helped and assisted healing the outer wound of physical illness I had manifested. The inner world and the outer worlds mirror each other. Body, mind and spirit all work together to bring balance and health: or, they work against each other and bring disruption and illness.

The following poem has come to express for me the positive aspects of this death process that I experienced. I believe it also describes the continual challenges of the mini deaths we must go through each day in order to continue changing and growing in positive, healthy, ways.

Letting Go

To Let Go is not to stop caring,
It's recognizing I can't do it for someone else.
To Let Go is not to cut myself off,
It's realizing I can't control another.

To Let go is not to enable,
But to allow learning from natural consequences.
To Let Go is not to fight powerlessness,
But to accept that the outcome is not always in my hands.

To Let Go is not to try to change or blame others,
It's to make the most of myself.
To Let Go is not to care for, it's to care about.
To Let Go is not to fix, it's to be supportive.

To Let Go is not to judge,
It's to allow another to be a human being.
To Let Go is not to try to arrange outcomes,
But to allow others to affect their own destinies.

To Let Go is not to be protective,
It's to permit another to act their own reality.
To Let Go is not to regulate anyone
But to strive to become what I dream I can be.

To Let Go is not to fear less, it's to love more.
Anonymous

Letting go to this place of aloneness within me was a
pivotal point in surrendering to the next stage of struggling with the father. To begin to listen to one's own inner
source of information is the key to getting through both the
struggle with the father and the mother within us. Without knowing how to access our inner wisdom, we are
constantly going to others for advice, decision making, and
approval. This need for authority in women actually goes
back to the images from the story of Adam and Eve. When
Eve followed the serpent's advice to eat the apple of

knowledge and truth the result of this action was that all women in the West tended to be labeled by men as the gender that will cause the most trouble.

Since Eve's time, women have been labeled the bad person, the bad girl, the bitch, the witch, and have been warned to not step out of line again. Eve was also told that she was so bad that she was only to get knowledge from Adam, a man. We women have forgotten our inner sources of wisdom for advice and direction because we have been encouraged not to listen to this different kind of truth that is unique to women. A major lesson for me as I entered this "nothingness," or alone place that the illness took me into, was the importance of reclaiming my essential source of inner wisdom and direction as a woman. I think that a very personal and practical way for women to break out of this history of domination, is through reconnecting to silence and being alone. We need to touch the silence that teaches us the truth of ourselves, and we need to break the barrier that lets us once again be comfortable in being alone in order to feel our own strength. By reclaiming silence and aloneness we will understand both what we've held down in ourselves, and what the cultural system has held down in us, so that we can begin to change the way we live our lives.

In her book, *Making Our Lives Our Own,* Marilyn Mason suggests, in order to grow up you must trust oneself enough to know the kind of person you are, experience your feelings and voice them, be responsible for your life and connect to your spiritual self. She says that women usually don't stroll into maturity. She believes that women are catapulted into maturity by a drama that challenges old views. These "dramas" are such things as divorce, widowhood, loss of a job, health challenge, discovery that a child is addicted, etc. Women, she says, face *six challenges* in learning to feel like adults. The first challenge is *leaving home.* A woman must define herself separate and apart from parent expectations. The second, *overcoming shame,* means women should stop feeling responsible for everything. In the third challenge, *forging an identity,* women need to define themselves as outside their culturally prescribed roles. They can value the roles of mother, wife, and such but women need to go beyond them. *Integrating sexuality,* the fourth challenge, means being sensual and letting go of the fear of sexuality so that the negative part of being used by it doesn't shut us down. The fifth challenge of *claiming personal power* is knowing and trusting the little voice inside of us as women that begs to be heard. The last challenge is *finding our creative spirit.* This challenge, Mason says, is a spirituality of believing in something greater than ourselves (and not just a man!) that comes through us as beauty.

When we have the freedom to make choices, we can say no. "No" is an important word for women to learn to use. And "no" is the basis of working with the "witch mother." The other important word for women is "community." In community with other women, anything is possible. Women who have power and influence need them to help other women along in the process of change and growth. Most of all we need to mentor and support younger women. Together, we empower one another. But saying "no," being in community, and supporting other women to find their own personal power will never happen if, individually, we aren't willing to surrender to the battle with the "witch mother," and heal the "nothingness" we feel as women. As women we often think we've finished our "deaths" when we confront our mothers, and worthlessness as women, but in reality the biggest battle is still ahead of us. I was shocked with the next step I had to take.

7. Surrendering To The Shadow Father

As soon as I had gotten more clarity about my "witch mother," I immediately had an experience that related to the masculine within me. To set the stage for this encounter let me first describe what preceded this experience.

I had been blessed with meeting a woman healer. Mary had lived for many years in the mountains and had worked for years with native American healers. She had been trained, among other things, as a Reiki healer, and decided that it was time for her to move to town and use her healing skills with people. She not only had the ability to heal with her hands, she was a woman who had also deeply healed her own soul. Because of her own soul healing she had been called by Spirit to heal others, and was totally dedicated to the art of healing. Reiki had became an integral part of my healing process; this was not the traditional medical model healing but was the healing of the heart. I found that I needed both kinds of healing.

When I came to Mary for a healing session, she not only laid her hands on me for an hour and a half, but under the direction of her intuitive insights she helped me to gently go deeper inside myself. The healing warmth from her hands, and her gentle caring, was precious to me. When I first came to her for healing, I barely had the energy to walk down the stairs to her healing room. In fact, the first few visits David had to carry me down the stairs and lay me onto her massage table.

When I first lay on the table she would prepare both my body, mind and spirit with a silent ritual process. Gently she would place her hands on my body at exactly the places where I was hurting. As the heat emanated from her hands into my body, a feeling of peace and stillness would begin to relax me. At times I would go into a deep trancelike sleep, and when I awoke I felt deeply rested and more energetic.

During one of these healing sessions, after a time of giving me energy through her hands. She asked me to place my attention at the base of my heart and experience what she called, my Soul Being. As I followed her suggestions, I was shocked and frightened to experience a large, dark, luminous male figure right in the center of my chest. I felt weighed down by the fullness of the dark figure, and completely overwhelmed by it. As I described my experience, she encouraged me to ask the figure who it was and what it wanted. A thought flashed quickly through my mind and I said, "I know who the figure is, it is my male shadow side."

My mind had spoken faster than my understanding: I didn't know the meaning of "my male shadow side." I did know that a shadow was a dark, vague, indistinct form which is cast upon a surface blocking light. But I didn't understand what the "male" part meant. I felt confused not only about my unconsciously spoken words but also about feeling the figure's weight on my chest. For days after this session with Mary, I tried to make some sense of the dark male figure.

A shadow, of course, is very much a part of us as it follows us around, but we never really get to know it. I reasoned that the image and the message to me must mean that there was a dark male part of me that I was not aware of, and that it seemed located in my heart and soul. I was taken aback with these thoughts because, until this time, I had been struggling and battling with the female influences on my illness. I began to wonder what the male influence had to do with it. Like the "witch mother," did this dark, luminous male have a part in keeping me from getting better? As the days went by, I noted a series of dreams that I began having about the dark figure. The dreams helped to expand, clarify, and explain the mysterious characteristics of this male shadow side.

My first dream was about four black men. *I was walking down town, and as I walked by these four black men, they grabbed me and I became terrified. I called to the people who were passing by and I looked them right in the eyes and begged, to them, "please help me." But no one helped me. Then the police came and that was the end of the dream.* I believe this dream was saying that I had an incredible fear of this shadow, or dark part, of me. It had grabbed me and taken over my life. The fact that no one would come to my aid made me feel helpless and incapable of helping myself. Finally, help came in the form of another male authority figure — the police — which represented another patriarchal or male structure that had influence over me. In this case, saving and protecting me.

In the next dream, *A snake was going up my vagina head first, and I had David pull it out by its tail.* I interpreted this dream as saying that what happened to Eve in the garden of Eden was the same thing happening to me. The snake urged her to eat the apple from the tree of knowledge of good and evil. As she ate the fruit and got the knowing of good and evil, she was pulled away from the tree of wisdom by the man. I believe my generative and creative qualities are being pulled out or diminished by the male part of me. From this dream I began to touch the tremendous anger I have for letting this unconscious, dark masculine side of me, control the essence of me as a woman. As I got deeper into the anger, I began to realize it just wasn't personal anger, it was anger for what women have suffered in male-dominated societies for over 5,000 years.

These dreams touched my deep fear of being taken over and abused by men. As a woman, I did not want my body, my thoughts, or my mind to be owned by a man. I didn't realize, however, that I was taken over by the inner man as well. As I continued to record my dreams and write in my journal, I realized that I had been playing the role of a man in my life. I recorded some facts that hinted at playing the role of a man such as being called Patrick by my father as a child. The shadow of the male was cast upon me early, through the power of a boy's name. And, again when I decided to go to college, my parents encouraged me to get an education in something that was practical and that would allow me to make money like a man.

And, now, rather than becoming a housewife with children and a husband, I was out in the world earning a living, just like a man. When I was in my twenties and single, I had a lifestyle similar to a male bachelor. I was also making good money so I had the flexibility to be very independent; I was free to do what I wanted and to travel the world by myself. By the time I was thirty I had traveled over most of the continents, dated numerous men, been wined and dined in fancy restaurants, and bought my clothes at the best stores. I had developed a lifestyle most people would envy. Although most of my friends were getting married and having children, I told myself that I was busy trying to find the "right" man.

In my thirties I taught at a college and felt on equal footing with the men teachers. In fact, I charged my male superior before the administration for his ineptness. After leaving teaching, I had started my own consulting business. As my business grew and evolved I was brought into corporate settings, matching my energies with high-powered men and women in business. I remembered taking courses on how to run a business, how to establish goals and objectives, and, taking top sales training and time management courses as well. I was out there in the world to make my mark on it like any man would. I realized as I wrote these things in my journal that I had definitely lived a man's life rather than a traditional women's life.

As the days went by other dreams about men surfaced and I kept asking myself, "Was I really like a man? What did it mean for me to be like a man?" As I lay in bed remembering my old lifestyle I realized how radically my life had changed over the past year. But had I really changed? Because of the CFIDS I was no longer being driven by my work, or the male system, to compete and prove myself as successful. But, in some strange way, was I being driven by the illness? Now I had to question, from the dream material I was getting, whether I was trying to heal myself with the same male model that I had used all my life. Was the experience of the male coming to me as a shadow, a message, that I was unaware of how much control the male part of me was dominating even my illness? My healer friend said, "Patt, do you know what you have done to yourself? You have given the keys to CFIDS, and it is now running your life." I had thus allowed myself to be controlled once again by something else, something other than me. That was hard to hear.

The illness had forced me to live a much softer, calmer, "laid back" life style. I disliked this style of life, however, because it was the direct opposite of the style I had carved so comfortably for myself. My old style was to push, no matter what. But the more I looked at this old style, with its intense time schedules and focus on high stress productivity and the like, the more I realized it mirrored the whole authoritarian male structure. My life seemed much different now, sick in bed, except for the fact that I had given the keys of control over every single facet of my life to a new authority, Chronic Fatigue Immune Dysfunction Syndrome. The illness was now my authority; I was allowing it to control and run my life. I had moved from the structure of the outside male societal authority to a body/mind structure that urged me to relinquish my power to it.

I began to notice that when I had pains in my body I would naturally push them aside, ignore them, and they would simply get worse. My body was talking to me but I wasn't listening. But, just like the male-structured lifestyle, wasn't I supposed to keep to the corporate goal and not deviate from the path no matter what? In fact, for years I had paid no attention to my body when it hurt or got sick. Rather, just like everyone else I knew, I drugged it so that I could carry on with my work. Lying in bed day after day, though, I noticed that my automatic response of not regarding body signals began to change. Instead of disregarding pain, I started to pay attention to it and consciously focus on it. An amazing thing happened. The more I gave the painful part of my body my full attention, I noticed that the pain would shift and reduce a little bit. Whenever I slipped back into the old male style of disregarding the pain and not focusing on it, the pain would increase and I seemed to get sicker. The more I gave it my attention, however, the more it continued to reduce.

As I became more conscious that there was a male way to do things, and though my experimentation of focusing on my body pain, I began to believe that there was clearly a different way for a woman to do things. Although this may seem obvious, I had unconsciously lived with male values and attitudes as a shadow part of me for so long, this notion of female energy came as a distinct, new revelation to me. And I found I was making an energy shift from the way a man would do things to the way a woman would do them. For example, if I made a goal and really tried to achieve it, I would physically feel worse. For example, as I began to feel better, while I was under treatment at the Clinic, I purchased a knitting machine. I was determined to make a sweater in just a few hours so I pushed myself to make the deadline. The more I pushed to finish the sweater within the two hours, and, the more mechanical problems I encountered learning to use the new machine, the sicker I got. As I missed my two hour deadline, I got more ill and spent the next few days in bed as a result. I came to the realization that this kind of pushing energy was not wholly feminine. Knitting was a traditional feminine task but I was attacking it in a masculine high-productivity, controlling manner.

Right around this time I got a call from a girl friend. She was a highly paid commercial real estate saleswoman. As we talked she told me that she had been fascinated with her lover's comment that she was both highly masculine and highly feminine because, she could be on the phone making a big real estate deal, and the next minute in the kitchen making muffins, and, then, painting her face with makeup to greet him.

I was really struck by our conversation. I begin to wonder, given my frustrating experience with trying to control the sweater machine, whether she was really exhibiting equal masculine and feminine energy. The more I thought about what she had described herself doing, I came to the conclusion that she had no idea what it was to be feminine. Baking muffins or putting on makeup may be what women do, but she used the same "go get 'em" energy push to make the muffins and put on the makeup as she did to make the real estate deals. What a big insight this was for me. Being feminine may be something different than "doing" feminine things. I wondered, "What is it to be feminine? And further, does the masculine part of us act as the shadow, and, thus, not allow the light of the feminine to shine?"

What was this feminine energy, or feminine way of doing things, that was so different from what I had been taught? I began to feel anger toward women who exhibited what I called the "male energy." These women seemed to be competitive, cold, and aggressive. They were acting like men. Suddenly, they turned me off. Since I had many women friends like this, my anger surfaced at a lot of people. I especially didn't like it when I discovered that I was just like them.

I remember asking a male writer friend of mine what he thought the feminine was. He suggested that, for the answer, I should observe my new female, Maltese puppy, Shanti. "She will tell you," he said. I thought this a far-fetched notion. But the more I watched Shanti, the more insight about the feminine I began to get. Shanti was incredibly loyal to me. When I scolded her for something she did, she still came back with loving, heartful attention to me. Her joyful spirit lifted me when I got depressed. She would cuddle with me and lick my tears when I cried. She seemed to always intuit my condition and respond fully to me. Her high feeling and total devotion and comforting of me seemed to hint at what might be qualities and energy of the feminine.

During this time I started reading *The Pregnant Virgin* by Jungian therapist, Marion Woodman. She writes about why women have taken on so many characteristics of men and have rejected their feminine side. Her book helped answer the question, "Why does the masculine act as the shadow, not letting the light of the feminine to shine?"

I was shocked as I read descriptions that fit me. She

described how women reject their mothers early on in life because they see the mother as powerless in our society. One of Woodman's clients remembers that as an infant she looked up at her mother and didn't see any power in her eyes. At that moment, Woodman suggests, the infant decided that her mother is not the parent she will emulate. She chooses her father to idolize, follows his values, and projects her life onto his. Woodman writes,

> *The woman who has been a "Daddy's girl," for example, has seldom if ever experienced her "dark" side, her rage and jealousy, lust and ecstasy. Alienated from her body, she does not know the magnificent energy that is blocked from consciousness, so blocked that it rarely manifests . . . Body work accelerates the process and creates a strong container for the ego.*[1]

When a woman abandons the mother and chooses the father, she can lose touch with her feminine energy, thus also abandoning her emotional base and awareness of her female body. Unaware of her body she is not conscious to release body blockages which may result in dis-ease.

Ann Wilson Schafe's book, *Women's Reality; An Emerging Female System in a White Male Society,* also helped me understand the concept of the male shadow. Her ideas about the impact of the father on a daughter opened me to the core feelings about my own powerlessness as a woman, and my desperate drive to get power. She believes that the father, no matter how bastardly or how loving, whether he is home much or not, is the prime focus and example for a child. The child begins to emulate the father, not just as a person, but as a symbol for something they perceive they want. In our society the father has the power. Good or bad, successful or a bum, the man is prized in our society.

We, as little girls, go through a lot of circumstances that teach us that to survive we have to take on the male part and reject our feminine, often to the point that we lose knowing what the feminine is. We want to be on the winning side, not the losing side. We don't spend a lot of time even thinking about it. As girls, we simply notice the dominance of the male figure all around us. Our fathers were our key power model and we took on our particular brand of masculinity from them. If the father was successful we took on that brand of male success. If the father was dysfunctional and inept, we also took on those male characteristics. Good or bad, we choose the male characteristics to survive.

According to Ann Wilson Schafe, women

> get their identity externally from the White Male System and that the White Male System is necessary to validate that identity. Therefore, challenging the system becomes almost impossible. There is a direct correlation between buying into the White Male System and surviving in our culture. Since white women have bought into the system the most, they have survived better than other groups both economically and physically although they do get battered and raped and mutilated (for example, through unnecessary surgery.) They have had to hide and/or unlearn their own system and accept the stereotypes that the White Male System has set up for them. . . . Economic and physical survival have been directly related to accepting and incorporating the White Male System.[2]

Wilson goes on to suggest that there are four myths of this White Male System. First, the system believes that it is the only system that exists; second, the white male system is innately superior; the third, it knows and understands everything; and, the fourth, everything is totally rational, logical, and objective. The problem, she suggests, with this limited, linear, left-brained thinking, is that it causes a lot of stress to always need to be number one and superior.

I am convinced that men, as they are forced by our culture to adhere to this system, never get to grow up. Emotionally they remain like little boys. The white male system in our culture puts the pressure on them to be successful, make money, compete, and prove oneself. This creates intense expectations that few men can meet and probably accounts for so many heart attacks, strokes, high blood pressure, and ulcers suffered by males in our society. Now that women are following in the footsteps of men so closely they, too, are dying from the same diseases. While reading both Woodman and Schafe, I began to wonder how our society got this way, and whether it had always been this way. In thinking about how our society had became controlled by the masculine system, I remembered reading the history of the Paleolithic and Neolithic times.

As I reread this material from *The Chalice and the Blade* I realized that I fit into the pattern of a typical dominator society family member. My mother's role was oriented around the primacy of the family, and servicing the needs of the family. She played the role of the subordinate. In this position, her needs would be fulfilled as she played out this role. My father was a workaholic. He was always working at the store. The only male model I knew was that of the man of the family constantly working and away from home. I noticed that our meals and our life revolved around him; I also noticed that my mother was not happy with the routine. She complained about his long hours and his constantly being late for dinner.

Most women in our society, whether they themselves work or not, often believe they have no purpose in life without a man. Women have come to accept, through experiencing this male-dominated culture, that they can't feel whole without a man. Over the years, however, this focus on a man to give purpose wears thin on a woman. A low-grade depression can form in us, along with anger and bitterness. There is depression and anger because our self worth as persons and as women is so deeply diminished. Dissatisfaction surfaces in many forms. There is no doubt in my mind that many women in our society are very angry, and hold enormous rage that spills out on others or on themselves, often in inappropriate ways. No one can be in an inferior and in second-best position for a long time without having negative feelings.

I also shared no close emotional or inner world of fantasy or imagination with my father. Nor did we share much about either his or my daily activities. We did not share our dreams or much play. Marion Woodman suggests, in *The Pregnant Virgin*:

> *If her father accepts her inner life, then they genuinely share the eternal world of the creative imagination. Its values become her reality. Quick to recognize the illusions of the temporal world, she sets her sights on what is authentic, often becoming a veritable Cassandra, outcast by both her peer group and her parent's friends. . . . If her father is not mature enough to value her for herself, but consciously or unconsciously, forces her into becoming his star performer, then her trap is a very different one because it involves his rejection of her reality. Unable to recognize her own responses, she simply relinquishes herself to trying to please Daddy.*[3]

Like the little girl Woodman describes, my inner world

wasn't valued by my father. Instead, I became his little star. I realize that many of the things I did as a little girl to get his attention pushed aside what I really felt and wanted for myself. As Woodman says, I relinquished myself to please my daddy. I could begin to see, from both Woodman and Schafe, that I had taken on, unconsciously, the male-dominated model of how a woman is to act. But my question remained — how did all of this fit into my illness? I was reading this material during my hydrogen peroxide drip treatments. Reflecting back on this period, I believe I was exploring intuitively both what I needed physically, and what I needed emotionally and spiritually for my healing. These ideas of confronting the male-dominated culture we live in seemed far removed from my illness, but something inside of me said that they were connected. Day by day, alone at home, I kept following the lead of my intuition in order to explore what would come to me.

My dreams began to provide me with some further insights. I had two dreams that began to show the application of some of the ideas I had read about to my life. In the first dream, *I was soaking the labels from David's ties and eating them.* The first thought I had when I awoke from this dream was that I had taken on the values and attitudes of the male-focused values of consumerism and gaining status. But, soaking the labels before eating them indicated that I needed to soften some of the dogma in order to digest it. I may not describe myself as being as ruthless about getting ahead and having status (I might soften how I do it or say it as a woman) but I was "eating up" this pattern of life like any man is encouraged to do if he is to be successful.

In the next dream, *A 300-pound man was telling me that he was going to strangle me. I was manipulating, doing all kinds of things to escape from him. We were in a hotel and*

*I was going in and out of rooms to avoid the man. David was
present in the dream. I remember flying to get away from
the man. I woke up very frightened.* My interpretation of
this dream is that I felt like my power was being squeezed
out of me by the big, ominous male dominator society. My
way of surviving was to manipulate the dominator society
by being passive aggressive. I was always being defensive
in this male-controlled society and figuring out how to "fly
away" from difficult situations. I was angry at the position
I was in as a woman, but failed to speak out or actively go
against the dominator society. Rather, my protection was
to join them, as indicated in the first dream, and avoid
them as in this dream.

I've begun to see that, by definition, being married in our
society is being owned by a man. After many years of being
single, marriage became my shield. David was present
when the man was chasing me, but he really didn't do
anything for me. Marriage to David has protected me as
I've competed professionally more with men. But I haven't
confronted their criticism and intimidation of me. Instead
of confronting and disagreeing with men, or taking a stand
on an issue, or informing them of how their behavior
impacts me, I take flight and do not deal with them or the
issues. I "fly away," hoping that I won't be caught or
affected. From the fear in the dream, however, I had been
affected very deeply.

The more I thought about the material, read and worked
with my dreams, the more I began to feel the deep,
suppressed rage that I had held down for some 50 years. I
now knew that I wanted neither to "fit in" and "please
Daddy" in order to survive, nor to please a man.

I remember one day, when David returned from a
business trip, I met him at the door and screamed at him

about how much I hated being a women. I told him I was tired of the game of being told I was inferior, and how I wished I was a man. He looked at me stunned when I told him how lucky he was to be a white male in this society. I blasted him with all my pent up feelings, and as he tried to respond I stopped him with cruel cuts and biting criticism of him personally. I began to cry, and I sobbed uncontrollably for a long time. When David tried to comfort me, I would lash out at him with more anger and personal attack.

This rush of rage and hurt opened up in me the feeling of how really duped I had felt all my life in thinking that men would make it all right for me. In some unconscious way I thought they were like "gods," and because they were in control, surely they would take care of us women. They supposedly love us, and cherish us. But now, I began to wake up to the fact that I had been sold a false mythology. The world of equality as I had been taught did not work the way it was presented. The ideas of Betty Friedan and the other feminist women of the early 1960s about male domination had taken on a different meaning for me. I never really considered myself a feminist, but something was happening deep in my psyche that cut off the very meaning of who I was, a woman. I was not only angry, I was embarrassed and saddened by what was happening to me. The shadow was no longer a shadow; I was starting to let the light shine through it and this was painful.

The rage will still come up in me when I am having a conversation with a man and hear a sarcastic remark that's intended to put me down. I am clear enough now, however, to understand that men often try to punish women when they perceive them as more intelligent or successful. Often the sexual jokes about women are not just a "come on" but indicate men's inability to know how to handle their own sexual feeling for us. In masking their own feelings of intimacy through the joke, we get put down. We often hold back and make light of the negative remarks; we push the remarks aside so as not to upset the men. But men have upset women, and they continue to do so in unsuspecting situations.

For example, I was at an outing on a lake with a group of professional men and women. We were peers and colleagues. As we were talking, a dead fish floated near the shore. One women said, "I am down wind and can really smell the fish, let's move." A man near the woman interrupted her and said in a rather bold, angry, sarcastic manner, "No, it's Patt who you smell." I am always so amazed when men voice this kind of put down that I go into shock, and I make light of it. No matter how much I know that men need to put women in an inferior position, I still am in a dream world with the fact that men have anger at women.

Another interesting example of the put downs of women is how men want to relate to women's bodies. On the one hand they like the Playboy pinup and the porno film, but when it comes to really feminine aspects of our body they become hostile. Recently a model posed pregnant on the cover of Vanity Fair magazine and the press went crazy. The dominant male values, whether presented by a man or a women, surfaced in the heated debate. The cover was covered up at news stands, even though the woman's breasts were covered by her arms. In the picture one saw the profile of a beautiful, round pregnant belly. Does something in our male-dominated society make being pregnant embarrassing? Is pregnancy unpresentable in public? Is pregnancy viewed similar to menstruation, as a "curse"?

As women, one of our gifts is to birth life. But in many

ways the male-dominated culture has made birth into a baby machine. In some strange way we have made the "baby machine" something bad and inferior. Because the gender equality remains neglected by men, I don't think the women's movement over the past thirty years has changed the underlying feeling between men and women. If anything, the tension, the power, and the control is even stronger. In most ways men are still winning the power game, and we as women are still not true to ourselves. Ann Wilson Schafe suggests:

> *Because our position in this culture is so shaky, we have learned to lie. We lie to men and to other women, but mostly we lie to ourselves. We lie about who we are and about what we want and need. By learning to lie, we feel that we can carve out a niche for ourselves, but what this really does is to intensify our isolation and sense of not belonging. Once we start being honest with ourselves and with other women, our feelings of isolation lessen. Our cavern begins to shrink and fill up.*[4]

I believe it is difficult for us, as women, to really confront the destructiveness of a male-dominated culture on us just because of our gender. Yet, today, all over this planet horrible and unspeakable things are being done to us, just because we are women. Not for personal things we've done, but simply because of our gender of being female. For example in Islamic countries, husbands can divorce for any reason; women live behind a veil in public; women may travel only accompanied by a husband or a male blood relative; and women cannot work outside the home or drive a car. In Africa, 180 million women have been given female circumcision-mutilation of the external genital organs. This old rite of passage was intended to ensure that young women not stray and that they remain desirable wives. This situation has caused life threatening infections and has led to painful intercourse, infertility, and difficult childbirth. India has a tradition of dowry deaths — if the woman does not bring enough money to the marriage, she will be burned. In Israel 10,000 women known as Agunots are not given permission to divorce. In Brazil men sleep with many women; if a woman does the same with men this is considered adultery and she will pay with her life. In Asia, if by examination the sex is detected to be a girl, the woman will have an abortion. In Bangladesh, female children are breast fed a shorter period and given less nourishing meals.

There is a demeaning power that men have over women. Since men are the authority, they can abuse women at all levels of life. For example, rape is increasing in U.S. at a sky-rocketing rate; rape is now committed every six minutes. Rape is just a more extreme form of the anger and abuse often heaped on women in our society. Women also are thought not to have choice about whether or not to have a baby. Again, putting down the feminine makes the female more and more subordinate; and, raising the religious issue on top of it I believe adds to the emotionality of the abortion issue. The interest that our nation exhibits regarding having babies and, then, not supporting the family — compared to other nations — is appalling. For example in Canada, France, Germany, Italy, Japan, and Sweden all women have at least 12 weeks of maternal leave along with 80% of normal pay by the government and/or employer. Some countries have up to 55 weeks of maternal leave at 90% and the top country is Finland which has 35 weeks of leave at 100%. The United states has 0 duration weeks of leave and 0 weeks paid at 0%. And also the U.S. has no policy on day care availability. What is the message to women here?

Women bring life on earth which is one of her greatest gifts, but when she must adapt into a system that doesn't prize or want her gifts; something is really wrong. I believe women must do something different than to become like men and to denounce themselves as women. This is deeply ingrained in us; we have been mesmerized into the belief system that women are not OK and that their abilities and qualities are not as good as men. Basically, most women have bought the package; it has been a successful marketing campaign.

I then return to the question: How have these ideas and notions and beliefs, of the male domination over women, influenced my illness? When I worked in the corporate world, I could immediately experience the dominator qualities when I walked into office buildings. In these buildings were people who did not express their feelings, being tight and rigid; individuals who did not relate with others; and, a mode of thinking that was highly left-brained, rational, and linear. You could see these qualities in the way people interacted, in how the buildings were laid out, and in all the things that were taboo to talk about. This environment was opposite to my natural style, but I pushed ahead to copy these behaviors — I became like them.

Trying to take on these qualities of impersonality added to my illness. Trying to be other than myself put more stress on my body than it could handle. Many of the women who are getting CFIDS are outgoing, active, assertive, highly talented, and creative. They are successful by the white male standards of the society. What we may be seeing with CFIDS, however, is the denial these women are choosing in order to compete in a male-dominated culture; this is the opposite of a woman's natural style of interacting and living. According to Ann Wilson Schafe,

> *Women frequently go along with the expecta-*
> *tions of the White Male System in order to win*
> *acceptance. Most of us do this in one of two ways:*
> *either we try to act out the White Male System's*
> *definition of the traditional" proper" woman, or*
> *we try to be "like men." The latter choice is*
> *especially common among professional women. I*
> *remember a time when the nicest compliment I*
> *thought I could ever get was that I thought like a*
> *man. Of course I thought like a man! I was very*
> *well trained in the White Male System, but could*
> *men think like women?[5]*

Schafe's question overwhelmed me. "What was it like
to think like a woman?" I had no idea. From my interior
world, all that I had was the image of the rage of the big,
dark, shadow of a man in my soul. What overwhelmed me
was the knowledge that I had become a man. Being like a
man ran my life, and made me behave the way I did. I had
bought into the patriarchal system, and, in so doing,
rejected the mother and became the father. The reason for
the loss of supportive female friends, because I focused on
competition with other men in the work place, now made
sense to me. Schafe again says,

> *. . .why I began an intensive study of women*
> *is that we normally do not like or trust one*
> *another. In general women feel relatively safe*
> *attacking other women. We are not dependent on*
> *each other for our identity, so what does it mat-*
> *ter? This ongoing antipathy has severely hindered*
> *the growth and maturation of the Female System.*
> *The White Male System has used its observation*
> *of women inflicting pain on one another to dis-*
> *count the Female System. When women say, "I do*
> *not like or trust other women" what we are really*
> *saying is, "I don't like myself." And this in turn*
> *can be expanded to "I don't like femaleness"... To*
> *be born female means to be born innately infe-*

rior, damaged, that there is something innately
"wrong with us."[6]

As these ideas sank more deeply into me, the more depressed I became. I could try to change and be more "womanlike" in my work and relationships, but I believed that I would still be treated as inferior. I had criticized my mother for falling prey to the male system and not being able to get out of it, but I didn't see how I could escape it, either. When I begin to realize that a major reason for my illness was that I couldn't cope with the male-dominated world I was living in, I hit my lowest point. I fell to the bottom of the abyss as did Inanna. Nothing made sense to me anymore. I felt trapped. There was no familiar ground I could stand on. I had made my descent. I was surrendering into the darkness of death. I was surrendering to the realization that my father, that this male-controlled culture had stolen from me the right to be myself, to be a woman. The "shadow father" seemed far more powerful than the "witch mother." Somehow I knew how to fight the mother. The father was too powerful. I didn't know what to do. I was frightened and I wanted to die.

Death is when we let go into the unknown. I was at that point in my life when I had no more structure and no more hope. I had seen through what was driving my life and I knew something had to change, but I didn't know what. I had come to the end of what I believed I could do about my situation. I saw no more future with my health or with my life. I couldn't go on like this and I wanted to die. I had lost all sense of the value of my illness to the rest of my life. Stephen Levine, one of the authorities on death and dying suggests,

How often, for instance, is one encouraged to
contemplate the aches and pains of the flu as a

preparation for death, as a means of melting the resistance to life? We seldom use illness as an opportunity to investigate our relationship to life in order to explore our fear of death. Illness is considered bad fortune. How do we allow ourselves to come into the courage that allows life its fullness?[7]

I had been trying to explore the psychological and spiritual implications of my illness so that I could get healthy again. But I hadn't used my illness to explore my fear of death. My whole disease pattern had to do with lying to myself about who I was, and of resisting my own nature. I no longer had any idea of who I was. I had played the male game for so long I didn't know how to change, nor did I know how to defend myself against it any longer. I was giving in. I was frightened, overwhelmed, and tired; I wanted no more of it. I blamed everyone involved in keeping the dominator system alive, especially the doctors who didn't know what was going on with me. They pretended they knew but they often gave me wrong information. The medical profession seemed to be the epitome of the white male system. I had had it with them as well as with my body fatigue, mental confusion, lack of spiritual interest, and my volatile emotions of angry, rage, terror, loneliness, and depression.

THE DEATH AND AWAKENING STATES

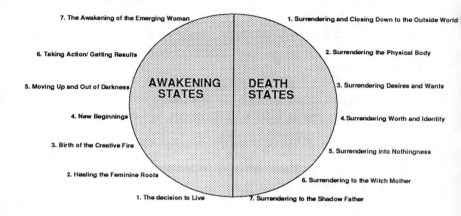

7. The Awakening of the Emerging Woman

6. Taking Action/ Getting Results

5. Moving Up and Out of Darkness

4. New Beginnings

3. Birth of the Creative Fire

2. Healing the Feminine Roots

1. The decision to Live

AWAKENING STATES

DEATH STATES

1. Surrendering and Closing Down to the Outside World

2. Surrendering the Physical Body

3. Surrendering Desires and Wants

4. Surrendering Worth and Identity

5. Surrendering into Nothingness

6. Surrendering to the Witch Mother

7. Surrendering to the Shadow Father

The Awakening: The Seven Stages Of Rebirth

In order to recover from my illness I was forced to explore some very dark parts of myself, psychologically and spiritually. Each of the seven stages of death was one level of surrendering after another to uncover the inward roots of my outward physical condition. As I reached the bottom of the abyss in the last stage of "surrendering to the shadow father," I came to the point that I didn't want to fight any longer. I wanted to die, and I was serious about it. This next stage of my journey, then, is about facing death and making that choice to live or die. It is documented that suicide is now one of the common causes of death for Chronic Fatigue individuals. I, like so many others with the illness, faced this dark shadow in my soul.

This next section describes that confrontation and the rebirth it took me through. Like the seven stages of death there are seven stages of my awakening. If one is willing and patient enough, the descent downward will always turn and take us upward again. It was my blessing that the turn came for me and I was able to go through the awakening of a new birth spiritually and physically.

The Awakening: The Seven Stages Of Rebirth
1. The Decision to Live
2. Healing the Feminine Roots
3. The Birth of Creative Fire
4. New Beginnings
5. Recovery: Moving Up and Out of Darkness
6. Taking Action/Getting Results
7. The Feminine Awakening

1. The Decision To Live

> *Who is prepared to die? Who has lived so fully*
> *that they are not threatened by imagining their*
> *non-existence? For it is only the idea of death that*
> *frightens us. It is the unknown that we pull back*
> *from.*   *Stephen Levine*

We live in a society that denies death. But what I found was that it is easier to die than to live. Death is confusing to us because it is so "hush-hush" in American society. In many ways talking about death is like talking about sex, we are both embarrassed and un-knowledgeable about it. From a mass culture point of view we spend billions of dollars in foods, diets and exercise equipment to keep the body young so that we don't have to face death. We have incredible fear about getting to the end of our life, and we avoid the thought of it. We have many unanswered questions about where we go when we die and what is going to happen to us. Psychologists and religious figures suggest that the unconscious, underlying fear of facing death actually stops us from letting go of our self constraints and really living life. Stephen Levine writes, *"The confrontation with death tunes us deeply to the life we imagine we will lose with the extinction of the body."* [1]

As I lay in bed day after day barely able to do anything or see anyone, I thought about the low quality of my life; it consisted of trips to the clinic for treatments of oxygen drips and then coming home feeling worse than when I went. I was either nauseated, had chronic low energy, or experienced feelings of depression. Life didn't make much sense, and more and more I welcomed the thought of death. I actively begin to feel that I wanted to take my own life. Several times I asked David if he would help me die. The first time he didn't answer me. The second time he said, "I couldn't help you do it, but it is your decision." In 1989 Susan Griffin, also suffering from CFIDS, wrote an article, *Canaries in the Mine* in which she shares, *"Now, at this early hour I have the same feeling again. It is not a feeling I have had with any other illness. Others with immune disorders have also spoken of it. One feels the world dying within one's own skin."* [2]

One day during this time, David sat down next to me, and very quietly asked me, "Do you think you are dying?" I said, "Yes I do." Then he asked me another very important question. "What is it that you haven't done in your life that you would want to do before you died?" I was amazed at how quickly my answer came. "I want to do something with music," I replied. I am not a musician, but I love music and I actually wanted to be a music major in college. In the 1950s, majoring in music was not the most practical thing to do to get a good paying job, so I majored instead in science. I paused and then said, "Before I die I want to experience the feelings I had in a dream where I sang. I want to do what my dream revealed to me." Two years before, and about six months into my illness, I dreamed about inspiring others through my singing. I opened my journal and read my dream notes to David.

> *I was waiting for my college girl friend to go somewhere. She did not come, so I telephoned her and the message was that she would not come. I felt left out. In the next scene I am waiting for her again, in a factory, and, finally, a young man comes to me and tells me he had just been with my friend. He gave me her phone number and some coins to call her. I called and she cancelled again. I felt very unloved, unwanted, rejected, and didn't feel good about myself at all.*

> *I was going to have to work singing in a club, but I felt dejected, and with low energy. I had on a new red and black dress and as I took off my red sweater I heard the announcer introducing me. The announcement made me feel good. The piano music started and I couldn't remember the words so the pianist started playing and singing; I then joined in after her. The words of the songs were something about having to have a vision of your-self to truly know who you are. It must be a vision, not something verbal, or some actions. I belted out the song and when I finished the place was packed. There had been only three people in the audience when I started. After the song I started talking about how our feelings are in the core of us; I then started to sing and wake up from the dream at the same time. As I was waking up I had the sense of singing for people who needed uplift-ing making them feel good as well as teaching people about themselves.*

After reading the dream to David, I got excited about the possibility of singing and teaching. He looked at me and said, "Why don't you try to do it?" He went downstairs and

I immediately began to think of the ways that I could make my dream happen. The possibility of fulfilling my dream lifted my spirit for several days. Then I began to talk myself out of it. As I thought of all the reasons why I couldn't do it, I got depressed again and began to wonder why I was getting so frightened about trying. The idea struck me that, by expressing myself and finding my own voice, I would have to confront the disease in my throat.

For a long time I had experienced pressure and tight-ness in my throat. When the doctor examined me he found the problem to be Hashimoto's thyroiditis, an autoimmune disorder which causes an under-activity of the thyroid gland. Situated in front of the neck just below larynx, the thyroid plays an important role in controlling the body metabolism. Could the fear and tension of not expressing myself, yet wanting to sing, be the inward cause of the outer disorder of thyroiditis? Was the under-activity of singing creating an under-activity of thyroid production in the gland? For years I had thought, "I am too shy to sing in front of a group. I am not a professional and I will be criticized." The other part of the tension was the deep inner drive to somehow express myself with music in my work. I remember a childhood book where the little girl's arms were being pulled in either direction. That was me. Maybe, I thought, my body really is communicating something to me. As *A Course in Miracles* says,

> *Healing is a result of using the body solely for communication. ...Mind cannot be made physical, but it can be made manifest through the physical if it uses the body to go beyond itself. . . A mind that has been blocked has allowed itself to be vulnerable to attack, because it has turned against itself.* [3]

Remembering how sick I'd been, and having the intense

feeling that something was missing in my life, the thought from *A Course in Miracles* validated and helped me take my thoughts to the next step. I thought to myself one day, "I just don't care what other people think, I need the music for my own enjoyment, my own fulfillment." The pain of not doing my singing was now more intense than the fear of doing it. People, I reasoned, would either like my way of using music or not, but I had to try to do it. Anyway, if I was going to die, what did I have to lose?

I told David the only reason I wanted to live would be to try out the dream in real life. We talked more and David gave me some ideas. I started feeling an old familiar feeling of creative excitement. It was the excitement of creating something that really interested me, and that was the results of my effort. I remembered Marion Woodman writing in *The Pregnant Virgin* about women in their midlife. She said if they did not find or use their deeply longed for creative talent they would die either physically or mentally, and emotionally, feel unfulfilled for the rest of their lives. Marion Woodman goes on to say,

> *In my experience, there is one very dangerous passover to be made with the creative woman. If she is in a mid-life crisis, has recognized that she has not yet taken responsibility for her talent and has lived a basically person-oriented or animus-dominated-life, she may suddenly reclaim her abandoned child and attempt a 180-degree turn with all the determination of the outcast about to come into her kingdom. Either the archetypal influx is too much for her immature body, or the ego is not sufficiently related to the body energy, or the psychic shift is too sudden for the body to move in harmony with it. Whatever the cause, there may be serious physical symptoms. It is as if the initiation rites that were not assimilated at puberty have now to be integrated before the rites of menopause can be endured.*[4]

I felt like I had always been a creative woman and I was at some kind of critical crossroad. I was serious about dying and I was serious about my music. And the tension between the two had created a very "serious physical symptom," to use Woodman's words. Was I experiencing some kind of initiation rites that I had never assimilated in childhood? Indeed, by taking on my father's views and values, I had left behind my desire to embrace music full time; I had become a practical "man-woman." But was I the truly creative woman that Woodman spoke about? It was clear that I hadn't taken responsibility for the musical talent that I had. When given the chance in college, I didn't let it mature or develop. Now I was faced with seeing myself differently and making a major shift in my life. I wasn't sure if I could "grow up" and make a mental shift about myself, but I knew I had to try. I began to have quick flashes of joy that I hadn't felt in years. The possibility of singing for others thrilled me. "Maybe," I thought, "this physical struggle is to help me reclaim what I lost in my youth." I began to look at a familiar quote from *A Course of Miracles* quite differently as I contemplated this notion.

> *I am responsible for what I see.*
> *I choose the feelings I experience, and I decide*
> *upon the goal I would achieve..*
> *And everything that seems to happen to me*
> *I ask for, and receive as I have asked.* [5]

To tell the truth, during the whole time I was ill I disliked this quote. I could not believe that I was creating my own sickness. But I didn't want to be sick. With the new perspective about singing, I realized that I had not been responsible to myself, but, rather, I had been responsible to my illness, to my fear, and to an authority that was outside myself. I know I am not happy when I place my attention outside of me. When I give my personal power to something outside of me I feel drained, confused, and have difficulty making decisions because I am going against my natural inclination. This, I thought, is similar to the auto immune diseases I have. It depends on where I am looking and to whom I am responsible. If I look at my inner wishes, I feel the excitement of the music and my dreams. Then I am responsible to that part of me, and I must trust it and go with it. If I look on the outside and see the fear of not being able to do what I want, or focus my attention on what people will think, then I will give away my personal responsibility and power.

One of the premises of our dominator society is to obey and look to it for one's salvation. If we don't accept its rules or play the game, we may be relegated to the bottom of the pile, to the lowest places in the hierarchy. Not just education, but the right school is important. Not just a house, but a house in the "right neighborhood" if you want to get ahead. We learn to obey at a very early age not just our parents, but our culture as well. Those who don't play the game are suspect; some reject the rules and become criminals; many remain at the margins, at the outer edges, of society. I always played by the rules. I played to be near the top. But one of the rules was that one would be excused from the general rules when one got sick.

When I got tired of playing by the rules when I was a child, I got sick. By being sick I got to be different, to be taken care, to not have to do the normal things of life for awhile.

In a flash, one day lying in bed, I got it. I thought, "This was it! I don't have to get sick to take responsibility for the direction I want to go in." As a child I got sick to get attention and to get some extra care and thoughtfulness. I was now in a situation in which I didn't know what to do, I didn't have a guidebook. I was trying to step outside the accepted cultural rules so I could figure out what direction to take. I realized in my case that the illness had forced me to stop so that I would either reclaim an old direction, of singing, and music, or probably, choose to die.

I think it is incredibly important for women to make decisions for ourselves. But before we make a decision, I believe we must also realize that "what I am and how I feel," is the most important thing to consider; it's not just a decision of "what do I do?" *A Course in Miracles* says that this ability to truly see ourselves comes in a form of recognition of some inner vision and the suspension of judgment about ourselves. If I look within and see the beauty of myself, wholly independent of inference and judgment, then I will be in a state of responsibility to myself. I can then get well by looking to myself for my own happiness. Looking inside of me and seeing myself singing to others makes me feel incredibly happy.

> *Deceive yourself no longer that you are*
> *helpless in the face of what is done to you.*
> *Acknowledge but that you have been mistaken,*
> *and all effects of your mistakes will disap-*
> *pear.*[6]   *A Course in Miracles*

I had another dream at this time.

> *In my dream, I was at comedian Steve Allen's*
> *home with another woman. We were talking to*
> *him outside. I said, "You are a man who doesn't*
> *have an office, but works out of your home." He*
> *agreed and was pleased that I was so insightful*
> *about him, and took time to notice him. He looked*
> *healthy, not old, without wrinkles. He had ma-*
> *ture, flared nostrils which I take to mean a*
> *frontier-type of person. As he left, I noticed that*
> *he was in a wheelchair and that he was going to*
> *an outside building. It looked like it was a recre-*

*ation building and he was going to be with his
wife and children. They were inside. It seemed
like they were having lots of fun. As we bicycled
away, I realized I had forgotten my potato chips,
the ones I like so much. We turned around to go
back and get them.*

The idea of being a creative entertainer like Steve Allen
represented something new to me. His having a handicap,
an illness, also seemed to match me. The feeling from the
dream was a comfortable connection with Steve Allen, that
he liked and approved of me. The male part in me is the
worldly musician and showman, but is unable to walk or
take the next step forward due to being handicapped. For
one thing, I did not believe that I was creative. But I had
once heard a Unity minister say that "we are created in
God's image and She created heaven and earth, so we
women are all creative!"

In *A Course in Miracles* we learn, if I am part of God, the
creator, and Mother Earth, the creator of life, then I believe
I am also creative. If I choose to make the outside world my
God, then I will suffer; If I choose, however, to make God
my authority then my gift is happiness. The *Course* also
suggests that I chose to give this whole view of the dominator system to myself; this was my gift to myself. I
listened to the world around me and convinced myself that
it was really true. And now I need to see the world and see
myself differently.

I know the possibility of having a creative life with
music was the pivotal factor that prevented me from
choosing to end my life. The switch from wanting to die to
wanting to live however, wasn't done in a day. It took time.
The movement from death to life was slow in coming and
it came to me quietly. But when it became fully conscious
in me that I wanted to sing and was willing to try it, I

stopped thinking about dying. One day I heard myself say, "I didn't really hear God's call to take me home. When I hear Her voice calling, then I will be ready to go through death."

What I think happened is that, like Inanna, I had to be stripped bare of old beliefs and let go of everything in order to get to the point, at bedrock, at the bottom of the abyss, where I was able to be touched by the Spirit of Energy we call God, and Goddess. I also felt that some part of me knew that I shouldn't let go of life any further, and that I needed to reverse my direction — I had reached bedrock and it was time to return to the surface and reawaken to my life.

I strongly believe that we are deciders, not doers. The actions we take, or the results of the decisions we make, will come in our lives after we decide. When I made the decision to live, I received three telephone calls within the next week that shifted my life. The first call was from a man who had built a hot tub for me years before. He also suffered from CFIDS and had recovered from it by using liquid oxygen. The second call was from a woman who said that her father had been treated with the oxygen drips in his arm at a preventive clinic. The third call was from a man who no longer had kidney stones after he stopped eating the foods he was allergic to. All three of these individuals recommended a preventive clinic that I had never heard of, located just one hour from our home. As soon as I made the inward decision to live, there was an almost immediate outward change, providing a way for me to choose to begin healing my negative physical condition. To do this I had to surrender to the overpowering control of the "Shadow Father," both personally and in the dominant culture. From a place of despair I had to abandon myself and be willing to physically die. This action permitted me to turn away from the abyss and start my upward journey to awaken a rebirth of a new identity, both as a woman and as an individual. Marion Woodman, in the *Pregnant Virgin,* affirms this process when she says,

> *For many women born and reared in a patri-*
> *archal culture, initiation into a mature woman*
> *occurs through abandonment, actual or psycho-*
> *logical. It is the identity-conferring experience*
> *that frees them from the father.*[7]

2. Healing The Feminine Roots

As described in Part III, the work with the oxygen drips and the diet was a slow and difficult process. Although I had made the inward choice to live, the physical struggle of living took tremendous effort and focus. Yet the process inwardly continued to demand my attention as well. The parallel effort between my outer and inner healing changed my life significantly.

As my body healed and I worked with my dreams, I noticed I was less angry at the "witch mother," both with my birth mother and the one inside me, as well as more open to male friends. I had a clearer mental perspective on things. As my emotions became more balanced, I was able to concentrate again; I found books and read about women's history. With thirty years of the feminist movement in our country, there is still very little "her-story" taught about women in our schools; we only hear "his-story." In the 1970s and early 1980s when I was teaching in the biological health sciences, I observed the women's department struggling to survive to keep women's classes open to women. Although I was interested and supportive of women's issues, I had done little reading in the field. I was now eager and ready to know more about the history of women's struggle to attain freedom and equality. I also talked with other women and saw many films about women and made by women.

From a western cultural point of view I tried to understand Eve's part in our creation story. This infamous event at the beginning of time offers clues, I believe, about our problems. From Eve eating the forbidden fruit, I believe women were then considered manipulative, devious, and subservient to men. I never quite understood why we got saddled with the total responsibility for this event. Why wasn't Adam given some responsibility in the situation? In her book, *Reinventing Eve,* Kim Chernin suggests,

> *By eating a food she was not supposed to eat*
> *she became responsible for the fall of man. . . .*
> *When Eve fell, the terrifying power of the God*
> *worshipped through obedience to his diet fell*
> *with her. In this sense: Eve was the rebel, the first*
> *woman to challenge the subjugation of woman in*
> *the patriarchal garden... For thousands of years*
> *women have had to adjust to a world created by*
> *men. Potentially capable of creating ourselves we*
> *are not easily at home in this world where woman*
> *may only become what man wants her to be.*[1]

As I read Chernin's book I was eager to investigate further back in time, and into other cultures, to compare the beginning views about women. I had read somewhere that there were new archaeological excavations and new scientific findings from old diggings that re-examined society from a gender perspective. *The Chalice and the Blade,* was written by a woman, Riane Eisler, who did a tremendous amount of research that can help us as women understand more about the unconscious patterns that we live by today. But, besides an analysis of how we got to this point in history as women, she also gives us the possibility of a different kind of gender relationship. A number of her ideas helped me as they form a solid basis for the next stage of my own growth and change.

Eisler shares her basic premise, that we, as human

beings since the beginning of time, have lived in two fundamentally different models of society. The first is a social system in which the power of the Blade is idealized. This is a society in which both men and women are taught to equate true masculinity with violence and dominance, and to judge men who do not conform to this ideal as "too soft" or "effeminate." This system of society also sees women as not fitting into this model as they too, are soft, weak, and subordinate. She calls the "Blade" society the *"dominator* model" to identify different cultures worldwide throughout history that adopted this model. What is interesting to note is that the dominator model of society can be either a patriarch or a matriarch because it utilizes ranking as its cultural criterion. Almost all societies on the planet today rank one half of us over the other half, men over women. It worships the power of the blade. Eisler states that the dominator system is, *"The power to take rather than give life. That is, the ultimate power to establish and enforce domination."*[2]

The second basic model of society uses the principle of linking rather than ranking. Eisler calls this the *"Partnership* model. "* In this model people are considered neither inferior nor superior to one another. This cultural model of Partnership takes as its primary value the life-generating and nurturing powers of nature. The closest image occurs in the Arthurian legends and is symbolized by the chalice or the Grail. The cup symbolizes the feminine image of receptivity to life. Eisler asserts in her book that there was a time when our foremothers and forefathers were in a partnership relationship without dominance or subordination of either gender.

Eisler presents the "cultural transformation" theory that proposes that the origin of our cultural evolution was one of partnership. After a period of societal chaos and cultural disruption, however, a pivotal branching and a fundamental social shift occurred, about ten thousand years ago. According to Eisler, "There appeared on the prehistoric horizon invaders from the peripheral areas of our globe who ushered in a very different form of social organization." These invaders of Mediterranean areas came from inflexible, male-dominated societies from what would now be northern Eastern Europe and the former Soviet Union. These people had hierarchical and authoritarian societies based on a high degree of interpersonal violence and warfare.

Eisler argues that the societal structure that one lives in fundamentally affects all human relations including our religions, our education, our institutions, our values, and all the permissible behaviors by which we run our life and run the world. These structures determine whether our society will be peaceful or warlike. This idea woke me up to the realization of the kind of cultural system in which I live. I had been so influenced by this domineering cultural structure that it had diminished my voice as a woman and in turn, had affected my self esteem, confidence, physical health, and life vitality. This was not an illusion, but a fact. I began to ask myself whether other women were struggling with this issue, too. I wondered whether men liked their role as the "fierce" dominator. But then I thought, "What about women, those who take on the dominator role? What impact was it having on them?" All my questions led me to more study.

What was society like before the bifurcation (this splitting between dominator and partnership cultures), and the pivotal shift towards dominator cultures on the planet? Archaeological diggings from the Paleolithic time, over thirty thousand years ago, have discovered some very different types of ancient societies. These important records from the site diggings have produced wall paintings, cave sanctuaries, and burial sites with female figurines. The emphasis of life by many of our early ancestors seemed focused on women. The records particularly show this in the context of giving and preserving life, and, in certain rites to bring about rebirth. From the female figurines found in the diggings, researchers discovered that the woman's body was used as an image of worship. Because of their ability to give birth and carry the life-sustaining powers, the female was valued. Also found were figurines in the combined form of animals and women, showing the connection with nature in their religious life. From these findings, scholars assume that Paleolithic people's views were that nature must be treated with respect because all human life springs from this source.

After World War II new evidence was unearthed that shed more light on the next period, the Neolithic period, about ten thousand years ago. These forebearers were the first agrarian communities in Asia Minor, South Eastern Europe, Thailand, and Middle America. The largest known Neolithic site at Catal Huyuk, in Turkey, is on thirty two acres. Only one-twentieth of this site has been excavated. Yet, the variety of artifacts that have been found are amazing windows into the life these people lived. Among the artifacts that have been found are wall paintings, plaster reliefs, decoration on vases in the form of birds, egg shaped stone sculptures which are thought to be symbols of birth, serpents and butterflies that depict metamorphosis, and large quantities of the round Goddess figurines made of clay. These objects represent an advanced religion of worship of a feminine deity. With this feminine focus of culture we find the birth of architecture, of community planning, of agriculture and stock breeding. The evidence shows an equalitarian society not marked by distinctions based on either class or sex.

A University of California, archaeologist, Marija Gimbutes, writes in her book, *The Goddesses and Gods of Old Europe, 7000-3500B.C*, that *"an equalitarian male-female society is demonstrated by the grave equipment in practically all the known cemeteries of old Europe."*[3] She also shows that these societies were matrilinear, so that the birth genealogy is traced back through the mother. Eisler summarizes the Neolithic time as a period when feminine-oriented societies based their structures on the *"theme of unity of all things in nature, as personified by the Goddess, as this seems to permeate Neolithic art. For here the supreme power governing the universe is a divine Mother who gives her people life, provides them with material and spiritual nurturance, and who even in death can be counted on to take her children back into her cosmic womb."*[4]

Something dramatic switched inside my gut after reading about these ancient societies. This ancient wisdom information gave me a new perspective about my "roots" as a woman. As a woman I am historically connected to a matrilineal society, that is, rooted in a female deity and functions with an equalitarian approach to life. For the first time in my life, it filled me with pride for being a woman. These ancient people realized women's gifts and knew it was essential in the operation of the natural system of life to sanctify women in order for life to continue to flourish.

I became increasingly interested in how, and why, this basically cooperative social organization had been destroyed, or changed. These were societies of people where there was no concentration of property in the hands of the most powerful men. It was a culture without the supremacy of males over females. And it held as its highest spiritual values the generative, nurturing, and creative powers of nature. What events created the fall of this kind of society?

Apparently, nomads living around the edges of these societies became envious of the resourcefulness of the neolithic people. These nomads apparently needed more grass and water for their herds. These roaming bands multiplied and spread out and began to disrupt the prosperity and rhythmic growth pattern of the feminine-based neolithic societies. There is evidence of a bit by bit stagnation and regression of these societies as they were destroyed by invasions, natural catastrophes, and dislocation. Generally, the nomadic bands brought with them a powerful caste of warrior-priests. A significant difference of these nomads was their worship of male gods. It is evident that the fierce warlike culture of these people was in sharp contrast to the societies that created the basic technologies for agricultural production, art, and a feminine balance with nature. It is believed that a warrior-priest class of hierarchical structures brought to western culture the technologies for destruction. The process of conquest was much more complex, of course, but warfare was the essential instrument for replacing the partnership model with the dominator model.

As I looked at the pictures from Catal Huyuk and thought about the kind of culture we once had on this earth, I wondered whether we could ever again create a partnership society. Could this evolution happen again? This time, could the peaceful, cooperative, and nature-based peoples swing the tides away from dominance and war? Could non-violence and inner strength overturn the war mongers? Could there be another partnership society? I was both elated and inspired with the possibility. After reading these books on prehistory, I decided to next investigate ancestors closer to home. I knew that the indigenous peoples of America had a more nature-based value and tradition. I wanted to see if these peoples would give me clues about the partnership culture.

When Mother Earth was newly born,
Her body green and fair,
When giant creatures walked the Earth
A Mystery was there.

In every native invocation
As humans found their place,
Your fragrance showed in every nation,
in every sacred place.

My heart feels you in stillness
though my eyes are awed to see
Your presence in the mountains,
On the lakes and out at sea.

In every ray of sunlight,
In each cloud and stone and tree,
In every creature on the Earth,
Great Spirit! Blessed Be!
                                    Sudeep Looking Owl

In the tradition of native peoples, the stories a person tells about his or her people belong to the storyteller rather than to those listening to the stories. Ann Cameron was honored in receiving stories from the Vancouver Island Indian women. She was then granted permission to share these stories. In most Indian traditions, women are chosen to memorize the family lineage and pass it on to the children. Cameron's stories tell of customs, folklore, and of the death of the matriarchal culture, destroyed by the European explorers who brought disease to their villages. The loss of the storytellers was directly related to this disastrous epidemic. The stories captivated me; I envied the bonding from the women's traditional rituals that I read about in Ann Cameron's stories in her book, *Daughters of Copper Woman.*

The Vancouver Island Indians had a strong and re-spected "Society of Women." Cameron says, "*It was inter-*

tribal, open to all women, regardless of age, social status, political status or wealth. No woman could buy her way into the society. No woman could inherit a position in the society." [5] This meant that each woman was invited to join and participate in their rituals. The "Society of Women" had what they called a circle where they would meet and discuss their problems. If a woman came to the circle with the same problem more than three times, the circle did not demean the woman, but rather said the problem again would no longer be eligible for discussion with the circle members. The woman then, had to take responsibility for her life decisions. There were also women designated as warriors who represented the "Society of Women" in important adversarial situations.

How women were initiation into womanhood was one of the traditions that fascinated me. The women's role was to teach all girl children the legends, songs, and jokes. They specifically prepared the girls concerning how to care for their bodies, for marriage, and, for pregnancy and childbirth. And very specifically they would be taught about their "moontime" or menstruation.

The process for the moontime was fascinating. When a women began to menstruate they would go into the "waiting house" where they would spend four days during their moontime. This was the time they would sit on the soft padded moss and let their menstrual blood go back to mother earth. As a community in the "waiting house," the women would pray, meditate, play games, and celebrate together their menstrual discomfort by massaging and caring for one another. Moontime was a major event in the life of a young girl. Cameron writes, *"After you learned everything you had to learn, and the time was right, and you had your first bleeding time and been to the waiting house there was a big party. You were a woman."*[6]

The "moontime" party was a gala event with every woman attending that the young girl knew. The women elders would take the girl into a dugout and dress her in water bird down, considered the finest of feathers. An older women would lead her to the water, followed by the community of woman. Then, everyone would leave and the young girl would dive into the water and swim home by herself. *"The People would watch for her and they would light fires on the beach. When they finally saw the girl they would start to sing a victory song about how a girl went for a swim and a woman came home. As she arrived at the beach there would be chants, a joyous celebration, and permission given to the girl to marry and have a family."*[7]

The end to this matrilineal society came to a screeching halt, and their world was turned upside down. Cameron writes,

> *Strange men arrived in dugouts with sails that smelled terrible and were infested with sharp-faced bright eyed creatures the like of which had never been seen on the Island. These men wanted water, and food, they wanted trees for masts, they wanted women, for it seemed as if they had none of their own. Their teeth were pitted and black, and their breath smelled, their bodies were hairy, and they never purified themselves with sweating and swimming, and they talked in loud voices. They wanted otter and seal skin and were willing to pay with things such as the people had never ever dreamed. People got sick and died in ways they had never known.*[8]

These explorers were very different from the men in their villages. The explorers didn't sing, dance, or laugh; they claimed that the Society of Women was the Society of Witches. These men put the children in schools where they were taught to be ashamed of their bodies; boys were taught that girls were sinful temptresses who would steer them away from their true path; and that the girl's moon time was a filthy unspoken event. According to Cameron's research, *"By the time girls were allowed home to their villages their minds were so poisoned, their spirits so damaged, their souls so contaminated they were not eligible for candidacy in the Society of Women"*[9] The backbone of the womanhood had been crushed and the women warriors died fighting, leaving no one to carry on the legacy.

3. Birthing The Creative Fire

It has been said that when a woman takes seriously what it means to be a woman, she is pulling on a thread that can unravel an entire culture. As I read the history about how life used to be with the bonding together of native women in their villages, I was incredibly saddened. I never had this experience of bonding with other women. Maybe a community of women is what I had been searching for. As far as I knew none of my friends had this kind of communal bonding either. What was missing in my life was a community of women exploring what it was to be a woman. I didn't want an intellectual or a psychological pursuit of how bad or terrible everything was. I wanted something spiritual, firmly grounded in nature, like Cameron described.

About this time, our daughter announced her engagement. I wanted to provide the missing link into her life between David and me, as parents, and her, as a married woman. This link had been missing in my life. I wanted to officially create a deep acknowledgment of the separation from us as parents, and the creating of her own life as a married woman. I wanted to ritually acknowledge her moving away from us, but also to root us together at the heart and soul level so that we could grow deeply together as friends in the years to come.

Weddings are really the only ritual we have in this society that act as a bridge between childhood and adult life. But for me weddings had been a family show, a sophisticated party bash. I wanted an experience to create a deeper feeling of love with Shellie. I wanted something intimate that would let us reflect on our past relationship, and establish new boundaries in our relationships. My dream was that she be released from us as parents so she would be free to develop her own power as a women, and, at the same time, be fully present with her new husband, Michael. I was determined to have an initiation for her as she began her new life.

I believe rituals can be very powerful. The ritual with Shellie was powerful; it was a ritual for both of us, and it gently rocked me into a new beginning.

I had a friend who was like the women ritual leaders that Cameron described in her book. I asked this woman to help me create a ritual ceremony for David, Shellie, and me. She had chosen the ritual site to be in her lush, green, forested garden. The four of us sat around a table with symbols on it representing the native American belief of the "four directions." She used her ritual skills in asking the right questions and performing a ceremony which moved us to a deeper understanding of each other. Our time together brought many tears, and it opened doors of communication that we had felt too uncomfortable to explore before, or, that we were unaware of what needed to be opened. Our friend spoke to us of the meaning of ritual and initiation into womanhood and then wrapped yarn around our bodies to signify the areas in which we were bound to each other physically, emotionally, and mentally. As we answered her questions, and talked about past times together, the yarn was unwound and the ties that would limit our relationship were burned away with a candle.

We were deeply touched with the honesty and thoughtfulness of what we experienced. Toward the end of the ceremony, I felt tremendous love for Shellie and was moved by an incredible insight. The insight touched and filled me with joy and tears. I knew that without being able to experience this love for Shellie, the insight would have been impossible for me. I felt down to the core of my being what a gift she was to me. My insight was that I wanted to ground and make prominent the expression of deep feminine qualities in the way we lived, just as Cameron described it for the Vancouver Indian women. I felt that my role in life was to somehow facilitate and make a better life for Shellie and for generations of other women to come.

Sitting with Shellie that day I could not miss the message or its challenge to me. My commitment was to help women become aware of their feminine nature; to help them know their own unique patterns of the feminine; and, to know the long history of women in order to choose to reclaim the fullest sense of their worth and strength. My desire was that I wanted the lives of future generations of women not to be imprisoned as women in the past had been. Even if I could not do all of this in my lifetime, I would make a beginning so that it could be carried on by others. I was very taken and inspired to touch such a deep note in myself.

As it was a new beginning for Shellie, so it was a new beginning for me. For Shellie, the excitement of a wedding and having a married life had always been her dream. For me the beginning was the birthing of my life's work. For Shellie, it was leaving innocence of youth into the stage of wife and motherhood. For me it was moving from the stage of motherhood into the stage of crone or wisdom teacher. It was announcement time for both of us. Both of us were blessed with a birth, and of course a death, an ending, and breaking of old ties.

From the ritual with Shellie I could see what breaking ties can do in our lives. I believe that going into each phase of our life without acknowledging the endings, and the new beginnings, keeps us asleep. That is why ritual is so important. It brings out our highest longing and gives us a vision of what we are to do. At this time in my life I knew I could only go in this direction toward life. There was no other way, but up and out of the dark.

4. New Beginnings

Before the earth there was only water that stretched as far as anyone could see. Far above there was a sky land, in which grew a great and beautiful tree. It's roots reached in the four directions and it gave out every sort of flower and fruit. The wife of the chief of this ancient sky land had a dream that the great tree should be uprooted. Honoring his wife, the next day the chief ordered his men to uproot it, but they could not and so the chief himself did it. Where the tree had been there was a giant hole, and as the wife leaned over to look in, she fell, only clutching some seeds and leaves as she went. Far below some swans saw the wife falling, and flew up and caught her with their wings. Since the woman could not adapt to the watery world the animals lived in, they decided to dive down and get some earth from the bottom but no one could do it except the humble muskrat. The muskrat swam down and swiped at the bottom, grasping some of the earth. When he came up, he put the earth on the back of the turtle, and almost immediately the tiny earth grew to the size of this world. As soon as the wife planted the seeds she had brought, trees and plants sprang up everywhere. Life had begun on earth.[1]

The Earth on Turtle's Back:
A Native American myth

Vision and insight. Ritual and deeper connection with others. All this is wonderful. But daily, we have to live our lives a step at a time. With my physical health slowly returning, I couldn't just run out and start preaching to women about what had happened through eons of history to women. I had more to work on before I could do that. But many threads and pieces were coming together for me now. The desire to sing and play music was strong. The vision to work with women was even stronger. How do I put those two things together in my life? In time I would learn how they would unfold.

From my readings I began to understand how the feminine got so diminished by being controlled and placed under the rule of the domineering male tradition. The personal insight gained from our ritual with Shellie, about my life purpose, convinced me more than ever that the system of thought that we live under is destructive to women. The results of this understanding increased my commitment to listen more actively to my inner voice. To keep listening to the culture as I had for fifty years didn't help me. Actually, I hadn't read newspapers, watched television or gone to the movies for over a year, at this point, because of my illness. Now I was going to make a conscious choice to focus on listening to something deeper inside me.

This listening helped me to take more control of my life. I believe that we have to cultivate this voice for both daily guidance and survival in our lives. Whether it is as simple as what to wear or a major business decision, listening for this inner guidance is vital to women.

In the documentary movie, *Burning Times,* there is a graphic display of women listening to their inner feminine, being receptive to the earth, and following the wisdom tradition of thousands of years of healing people. The movie describes the events in Europe during the time of the witch hunts. Over six million women were hunted down and killed by the Catholic church during the Dark Ages because they listened to their own intuition to make herbal remedies, deliver babies, and do some of the traditional nature rituals from the old feminine based religion. Although we say that women have intuition and strong feelings, there may be some memory in us that knows if we really return to trusting and acting on our inner resources, separate from the dominating culture, we could get destroyed, too.

In some sense I had no alternative but to listen to my inner feelings. If I didn't act on what my body, feelings, and soul were trying to communicate to me about how to get physically better, I could remain an invalid and even die. So, for me, practicing listening to myself was survival. This reverse action, taking direction from my inner voice rather than the cultural voice actually reduced my pent up rage. I wasn't doing anything intellectually different to reduce this intensity. It was just that I shifted the focus inside and made decisions from a different perspective. I noticed the inward nudges of my body. I would sit quietly and ask myself a question and slowly open my eyes, noticing the change of light or color intensity in the room as clues to the "yes" or "no" I needed. I would watch for the sudden intrusion of a thought about a person, or some image of something that I hadn't been thinking about. Rather than dismiss these "signals," I would stop what I was doing and pay attention to a thought interruption, or try to interpret the meaning of my body sensations.

I wasn't always accurate on my interpretations, but the practice of listening to all these different aspects of myself was what was most important.

Years ago I wished I had been given instruction and permission on how to mark my emotional boundaries so as not to be so pulled and jerked around by others' emotions. I have had difficulty understanding which were my emotions and which were the other person's. I wanted to please people so much that I took on feelings and problems that weren't even mine. I tended to let myself be dominated by another person's attitude or view of life, and I would give more to them than I could afford to, and still be myself. As I became more personally aware of the history of the dominator system and how it works, I took the blame off others for controlling me, and I became more calm and willing to say "no" to situations that weren't good for me.

I believe this shift in my thinking helped the physical healing process as well. If it is true that the brain and the immune system are in dialogue with one another, my dialogue was softer, less angry and not so defensive. It made sense to me that I didn't need to blame someone for what was happening in my life. I believe we are victims of circumstances only because we have been asleep and let it happen to us. Being conscious of the dominator structure I live under and how it affects every aspect of my life, lifted from me a great burden of putting the blame on my husband, my family my friends and the medical system. The departure from the victim position gave me renewed hope.

As I began to get more inwardly and outwardly balanced in my life, I realized how separated I was from women. I had lots of close friends, I thought. But when I got sick I found there were few friends I could count on for help and support. I had a lot of acquaintances but when the chips were down, they went their own ways. There was no glue sticking us together. I was just following the crowd too. I had followed a man's path out into the world. That brought me some satisfaction, but mostly I got confusion and frustration. It never quite felt like I was enough. I wasn't a man. This confusion and frustration ultimately encouraged me into a search for why women no longer have the powerful community that our history tells us we once had with each other. Women seemed rootless to me in some fundamental way. And I felt rootless, even though I had a house, husband, and friends. Kim Chernin writes about our homelessness very powerfully:

> *For thousands of years women have had to adjust to a world created by men. Potentially incapable of creating ourselves, we are not easily at home in this world where woman may only become what man wants her to be. To be homeless in the only home we possess? Rootless but urgently requiring a sense of roots?. . .So we* **invent woman in the image of man's image of woman.** *High-heeled and charming, we become what we are expected to be: docile and seductive, good listeners, eager to make a good match, we long to build our nest and nourish our young and care for our man.. In this form we come to know ourselves, a diminished and restricted being who pretends to be at home in the world men expound.* [2]

I started once again to do more research into my dreams, my own feminine nature, and to read more about women. Again, I had many questions. How have women changed in the 20th century? What has the social evolution of women been for the past 100 years?

As I read women's literature, I came to the conclusion that women have been making radical changes that need to be noted and taken seriously. I read a revealing book, *The Awakening,* by Kate Chopin in which she writes about women living in the southern United States during the early 1900s. I hadn't realized just how passive women were, just 90 years ago. I started to examine women's response to their circumstances in the last 100 years. In the past three generations women have been making giant strides. We have come through three distinct times or eras. I call these three eras the Era of the Passive Women, the Era of the Man-Made Woman, and the Era of the Emerging Woman.

These time periods also seem to represent three styles of how women behave and respond in the world. Women do not always fall into just one era, or style but may fall into all three. The determining factor depends upon the life style of the women and the pattern of the feminine she expresses. This will show the qualities and characteristics she embodies from each era. Women may fit into each era but with different intensities. I had never thought in this way about these evolutionary times for women and I wandered what era I fit into. As I focused my search into these three time periods, I began to create a model that would give a foundation of where women have been, who they are now and where they are going.

WOMEN'S ERAS

I. The Passive Woman's Era

She believes marriage to a man gives her identity, stability, and worth.

- She is protected and taken care of by this man.
- Her image is one of weakness and powerlessness; his is one of strength, and success.
- She is limited relative to making decisions, developing her potential, and expressing her creativity.
- Her role is that of caregiver not only to a man's physical, emotional, and psychological well-being; but to her children as well.

II. The Man-Made Woman's Era

- She is part of the traditional male world.
- She tends to become a workaholic; taking responsibility for everyone including company, staff, friends and family.
- Her personal relationships are often secondary to her work.
- She imitates the male role in competition, appearance, independence, and success.
- Her feelings are repressed, protected by a tough outer shield.
- She is devoted to the development of her outer potential.

III. The Emerging Woman's Era

- She connects with her feminine self through nature, her body, and her creativity.
- She honestly voices her values and "follows her bliss."
- She will go against the male-dominated system for the good of the community.
- She is responsible to herself and partners easily with both men and women.
- She is self-contained, and protected by her inner resources.

In my research I also identified seven natural feminine cycles. These feminine traits evolve out of each stage as we grow up. Many of these feminine traits are considered weak and unimportant in our society, but they are our power, strength, and wisdom.

THE FEMININE DEVELOPMENT STAGES

The Idealizer Stage - (ages 1-5) The feminine traits of *bonding, intimacy, receptivity, vulnerability, and feelings.*

The Survivor Stage - (ages 5-9) The feminine traits of *intuition, time cycles, and rhythms.*

The Caretaker Stage - (ages 9-13) The feminine traits of n*urturing, softness, love, and openness.*

The Perfecter Stage -(ages 13-16) The feminine traits of *sensitivity, resonating with the body, and instinctual knowing.*

The Explorer Stage - (ages 16-25) The feminine traits of *following the natural individuation process.*

The Fighter Stage -(ages 25-42) The feminine traits of *individual and community leadership* .

The Integrator Stage -(ages 40s and on) The feminine traits of *sacred power and inner wisdom.*

As I clarified my view of the development of these feminine traits, first in myself, I noticed life events in each stage that may have either amplified the growth of my feminine traits or suppressed them. My next questions included: What kinds of women embody these feminine traits? What are their patterns? What feminine patterns mold us into certain types of women? As I read about women, and evaluated women I had known, I arrived at seven descriptions of adult women patterns.

THE ADULT FEMININE PATTERNS

The Professional Pattern - Qualities include ambition, being in charge, being worldly, and maintaining autonomy as well as perferring linear thinking, and being influenced by the male model. She is often her father's daughter, using verbal strategy, and integrating humanness and integrity. Her values include strong ethics and loyalty. *The shadow side:* Lack of attention to the body, repressed emotions, wearing a mask to impress others, and having conflict with dependence vs. independence.

The Sensual Pattern - Qualities include physical beauty, a sensuous nature, creatively talented, inspiring, and the symbol of femininity as well as being empathetic, romantic, warm, generous, and receptive. She chooses heartfelt relationships, she is often her father's daughter, and she is responsible, honest, and caring. The *shadow side:* She can be easily exploited, lacks personal boundaries, often manipulated sexually, avoids close relationships, often a player in the other-woman syndrome, and can be overwhelmed by feelings.

The Transitional Pattern - Qualities include instituting change and growth, taking risks, being sensitive as well as being inner-world focused, intuitive, and visionary. She is a mother's daughter, a healer, charming and can experience the dark night of the soul. *The shadow side:* She is unaware of her body, overwhelmed with too many possibilities, overly sensitive, and she often will choose to abort deep inner work.

The Outdoors Pattern - Qualities include focusing on a healthy body, being an athlete, active, adventurer, and competitive as well as being an independent thinker, instinctual, needing solitude, and protective of nature and animals. She is often a father's daughter, a character, has political interests, exhibits practical behavior, and is a woman's friend. *The Shadow side:* She is compulsive, addictive, a perfectionist, has tunnel vision, abuses her body, defensive and stubborn, needs approval.

The Family Pattern - Qualities include all aspects of childbirth such as bearing, nurturing, raising and educating children as well as creating safe home environments, weaving lives together, and caregiving. She is a mother's daughter, values children's future, family life, a solid foundation, and women's reproductive cycles. *The shadow side:* She lacks boundaries, is dependent, rigid in her beliefs, non-supportive, invasive and overprotective, responsible to others and not to herself.

The Community Pattern - Qualities include interests in power, authority, marriage, prestige, as well as being organized, confident, dynamic, dominant and having high standards. She is often a father's daughter, a leader, a gracious hostess, an influential wife, and a matriarch. *The shadow side:* She is aggressive, dictatorial and strict, critical, manipulative with power, malicious, and explosive.

The Soul Pattern - Qualities include the essence and the heart of each feminine pattern, gravitates toward sacred, tranquil environments, as well as living in the moment, central link to each feminine pattern, alive, rooted, joyous, gentle, kind, and consistent. She is the foundation and values the inner sacred marriage of the masculine and the feminine. *The shadow side:* She persuades others to follow her religious/spiritual path, distant and remote, totally focused on her inner life, and isolated from others.

5. Recovery: Moving Up and Out of the Darkness

The Mental and Soul recovery

As I did more research into women's history and women's psychology, it dawned on me that I was part of all this history, too. And so is every woman. I began to question how other women leaders throughout the world handling their diminished feminine qualities, their rage, their discontentment, their unequal status, and their health? I wanted to know what was happening to my peers in this respect I also needed to know why I got sick and why other women didn't get sick. I knew there were many women with immune problems. "Why," I thought, "did so many women suffer from these immune problems?" Was there a connection between their immune problems and their feminine patterns? Did they feel fulfilled as women? Or, were they the ones who had reached the top and said, "Is this all there is?" All these questions intrigued me. I was fascinated with the idea of finding out about other women's ideas, values, and behaviors. How could I find answers to my questions?

The plan that unfolded was to identify a small group of women and ask them the questions I had been asking myself. What would I learn? Wouldn't it be wonderful, I thought, if I had the energy to do this research and get the answers to help move myself and other women to another level of consciousness? Was it possible that I had gotten sick in order to change my direction, rethink my lifework, and untangle this information?" I didn't know for sure, but my own curiosity and the possibility of talking to other women about these questions motivated me. I felt much stronger now than ever before, even though I was still undergoing the various alternative treatments. I believed I could carry out this research. I had done academic research before, so I could do the mechanics of it. And, of course, I had no idea what the outcome would be. But maybe the project could also help to bring me out of isolation so that I could interact with my fellow humans again. I felt energized and excited—I kept remembering that the first notions about developing this project were those seeds planted when David asked me whether I wanted to live or die. And then, the strong commitment I had made at Shellie's wedding initiation, to help other women any way I could.

Physical Recovery

With the various types of treatments at the clinic, along with disciplining myself to keep to the regimen of a healthier diet, low emotional stimulation, and isolation requirements, my body was slowly getting stronger. I was able to concentrate more, and my ability to remember was better. My emotions were more balanced, and I was starting to regain my independence. But as good as this seemed, I knew I was not fully recovered because, I still needed naps and quiet times in the afternoons. My recovery was exciting but it wasn't complete. At this time, further tests indicated I had Addison's disease. When I understood that my adrenal glands were malfunctioning, but, that I also could do something about it, I choose to actively accelerate my physical recovery.

6. Taking Action/Getting Results

Taking Action

I began doing it! I started working on a research strategy My plan was to interview women who held leadership positions in various areas of professional life. I wanted first hand information about the feminine life from women who were "living and breathing" in a man's world Women who worked day in and day out with male values, male rhythms and male disciplines must have a clue about how to stay healthy And, perhaps, they could give me a greater perspective about why I had gotten so ill and how they stayed healthy. I was eager to learn the role they played in the development of the feminine and what Feminine Eras, Feminine Patterns, and Developmental Stages these women would fall into. As I began to formulate the questionnaire, thoughts and questions whirled through my mind. Why did I get ill and why did they not get ill? What was the quality of their backgrounds, their home lives, and did these qualities help them become leaders? What happens to their feminine selves when they work and live in a man's world? How do they cope? Do they notice any differences? How does this affect their habits, attitudes, behaviors, actions, and beliefs? How are women changing today? What kind of women are actively advancing womanhood today?

I contacted the perspective interviewees through friends and business associates. When I explained my research interview plan, I received a list of names which turned out to be a broad cross-section of prospects. I then contacted the women on my list and made arrangements to meet them in their offices or homes. The professions ranged from medical doctors, university professors, lawyers, business owners, corporate executives, therapists, organizational and management consultants, executive directors of non-profit organizations, corporate presidents, the director of a research institute, a film maker, a city attorney, and elected and non-elected political officials.

In my initial research I interviewed forty professional women leaders. In the interview I asked a set of questions about childhood, home life, perspectives on the feminine, their leadership position, their concerns and needs as a woman, and health issues I talked with each women for about an hour and a half. I also developed a set of questions entitled *The Feminine Assessment*. This is a 300 question assessment which includes questions divided into three sections: Feminine Era's, Feminine Developmental Stages, and the Feminine Patterns. Generally, this assessment was filled out during the interview or was done afterward and mailed to me. I made a commitment to each woman that I would make a follow up appointment to give them the results of the assessment.

As you read through the following list of interview questions try answering them for yourself.

Childhood Experience
What was life like for you as a child? What was your relationship like with your parents and siblings? What was school like for you? If you were writing your biography, how would you describe your childhood life?

Feminine

In your life experience, what was it to be feminine or masculine? How does the feminine act with men and with women? How does your feminine express your sexuality? What stands in the way of your feminine self? In your opinion (and experience) how does the feminine change as you move up the ladder of success?

Concerns

What drives you and where are you going? Who are your role models? What has it cost you to get where you are going? What keeps you out in the world away from your family? What troubles you? Do you have any unfinished business in your life? What is the wound, the sore place, the painful part in your life? What is your current frustration?

Leadership

Do you feel powerful? How do you want to experience more of your power? What is it like to be a leader? Are you making a difference? Is making a difference what you thought it would be? Do you feel whole? What do you see happening to women in leadership?

Well Being/Body

Do you have an exercise program and diet program? What is the condition of your body? Do you have a strong identity with your physical body? What kind of health problems do you now have, or have had in the past?

Needs

What kind of support do you need from people to make your life easier?

The results from the interviews

As I evaluated both the interviews and the individual assessments, I found some interesting parallels in backgrounds, particularly family and home life. This is a partial list of the statistical information from the 40 women I interviewed.

Childhood Background

- 41% were from divorced and broken homes.
- 62% have had one or more divorces.
- 79% were father's daughters.
- 13% were mother's daughters.
- 62% of their fathers were emotionally warm.
- 24% of their fathers were emotionally cold.
- 24% of their mothers were emotionally warm.
- 62% of their mothers were emotionally cold.
- 48% of their mothers were sick, mentally, physically, or were alcoholics.
- 37% of their fathers were sick, mentally, physically, or were alcoholics.
- 31% were sick or sickly as children and have had immune problems as adults.
- 46% had early responsibility at home.
- 37% were over protected.
- 72% were outstanding students in school.
- 41% went to college.
- 41% went to graduate school.

In the feminine area:

- 86% listed feminine qualities. The feminine qualities most listed were: soft, loving, mysterious, caring, nurturing, intuitive, and sexy.
- 62% listed masculine qualities. The masculine qualities most listed were: strong, aggressive, angry, active, direct, willed, and driven.

- 75% knew what stood in the way of her feminine self. Some examples were: perceived as fragile, feminine interpreted as sexy, and taken advantage of.
- 75% knew how the feminine changed as she moved up the ladder of success. Some of the examples were: more vulnerable, tough, more confidence, compromise time with children and husband, self dependent, and expressed more of the feminine.

In the area of past and present concerns:

- 79% knew what drove them to get ahead and knew where they were going. Some examples were: to earn money, survival, achievement, to be the best, excitement, and develop a better community.
- 38% had women role models.
- 33% had men role models.
- 59% knew what the cost had been to reach their current goal. Some examples were: intimate relationships, stress, overeating, illness, no time for self, and no private life.
- 68% were aware of the wound or painful area in their life. Some examples were; relationship with mother, not being married, relationship with parents, no family, loss of energy, loss of friendships, and feeling unlovable.

In the area of leadership:

- 82% felt powerful. Examples of what made them feel powerful: influencing others, solving problems, tested inner strength, reaching goals, and sharing information rather than influencing others.
- 72% want to feel more powerful.
- What is happening to women leaders today? Examples; hard to get ahead with the "old boys network," burned out, spread too thin, going into

own business, let down by men, lonesome, and extraordinary demands to be competent.

In the area of physical well-being and having their needs met:

- 51% were on a diet and exercise program.
- 31% were aware of their body and their own identity.
- The most often voiced need: someone to take care of wifely duties.
  Second voiced need was: women friendships.
  Third voiced need was: a close male relationship.

I was captivated by the information I received, and quite surprised how these women fit into my three-part model of the different Feminine Eras, the Feminine Developmental Stages, and the Patterns of the Feminine.

RESULTS FROM THE FEMININE ASSESSMENT

Feminine Eras

What time eras were these 40 professional women in? How evolved were they? How were they keeping up with the times? I was amazed that as successful as all the women interviewed were, some were in the Passive woman Era. What were the areas in their life that kept them stuck there? The questionnaire criteria I used to evaluate the Passive, the Man-Made and the Emerging Eras were the manner in which they related to the following categories: time, relationships, commitments, sexuality, intimacy, friends, parenting, money, leadership, rules, communication, responsibility, process vs product, conservation, and healing. Of the 40 women interviewed:

- 13% were in the Passive Women Era.
- 58% were in the Man-Made Women Era.
- 10% were in the Emerging Women Era.

Feminine Patterns

When I scored the Feminine Patterns Assessment I was very surprised to discover only a few women scored high as the Professional Pattern. Rather, I found the top scores were much different, in fact, the Sensual Pattern took the lead. Of the seven feminine patterns, the 40 respondents' primary patterns fell into just four:

Professional Pattern	7	women
Sensual Pattern	14	women
Transitional Pattern	11	women
Outdoors Pattern	8	women

Why is it the women who work in a male-dominated world need, or choose, to be strongest in the Sensual Pattern? As I evaluated the data, however, I found that no woman is just one pattern. Each woman usually had three strong patterns, with the remaining four not scoring as strong. The following is an example of the strong three combination:

Sensual Pattern is #1
Outdoors Pattern is #2
Transitional Pattern is #3

The other four patterns had low scores, which meant that this group of professional women utilized these patterns less frequently:

Family Pattern #4
Community Pattern #5
Professional Pattern #6
Soul Pattern #7

The stories that unfolded as I asked my questions were fascinating. I wish I could have filmed each woman's face as she unveiled the secrets of her life. There was a powerful energy that radiated from them as they shared some of their most intimate memories, sad and poignant as well as happy and joyous. As their stories unfolded, each woman painted a backdrop of events that, together, indicated how her core feminine self had become diminished, discounted, and manipulated by the male-dominant culture.

After first returning and giving them feedback on their assessments I then immersed myself in each woman's story; I wanted to try to understand and get answers to some of my basic questions about the feminine in women leaders today. To examine the results of my research, I retreated to a small cottage we built next door to our home.

It was here in the cottage that I placed the many folders in a giant circle on the floor, arranged my favorite rocker in the middle of the circle and for days, sat reading and studying and reflecting. I felt overpowered by each woman's story. But I needed more than a statistical calibration in order to fully understand the feminine. I wanted to unravel a single golden thread from each woman's story and assessment which would identify the theme of her strongest feminine pattern. I believed that this thread had been intricately woven into the overall fabric of her life. What was the gift that each woman had to give? What were the teachings I could glean, from each feminine pattern? The golden teaching threads from the four main feminine patterns began to emerge as I sat with their stories.

I. The Professional Pattern
• Playing out family programs, for the sake of the family.
    1. To be strong like dad so he will love her; she seeks to emulate him and takes on the male value system.
    2. To act as the power broker between her parents, to

represent that power brokering out in the world.
3. To successfully represent the family in the world; often a cover for family problems.

II The Sensual Pattern

- Being responsible for others, and being responsible for another person; the pleaser.
  1. As a child, taking the role of surrogate wife and mother; playing the second woman.
  2. The dream that her father would take care of all her needs.
  3. Adapting to any situation to get ahead; getting what she wants with feminine sexuality.

III The Transition Pattern

- Plunges deep into self and develops strength to be more true to her own nature.
  1. Weak emotional base and feelings of being unwanted or rejected by mother.
  2. Defers to others and blocks own passion; power play with mother.
  3. Physical illness that often results from holding on to people and on to situations.

IV. The Outdoors Pattern

- Reaction to mother's dominance moves her into nature or the male-dominated environment.
  1. Results of this rebellion is often the development of an individual's inner world.
  2. Nature is often used as solace and balancing of self.
  3. Finds it easy to match the vigorous energy of a man.

The other three feminine patterns were not as strong as these four, but they made a distinctive difference in the behavior and individuality of these women. I began to notice how the various combinations of all of the feminine patterns were integrated into the overall makeup, personality, and value system of each women interviewed. This merger gave each woman a "variation on a theme" and created a variety of individualized feminine patterns.

The following sampling of women leaders interviewed will offer a number of ideas and insights about the Feminine Patterns she uses, the Feminine Eras she lives, and the Feminine Developmental Stages she expresses.

The Professional Woman Pattern

ANN

AGE: 39
CAREER: Entrepreneur
ERA: Man-Made Woman
PRIMARY PATTERN: Professional
SECONDARY PATTERNS: Sensual/Transitional
DEVELOPMENTAL FEMININE STAGES: Integrator/
  Survivor
MEDICAL PROBLEMS: Food allergies, low energy
  syndrome, gastrointestinal

Ann is a 39 year old single woman, a strong, intelligent, efficient, professional type. To the outside world, she looks as if she has it all. Financially, she can bring in over $4000 a day from her own business consulting. In addition, she has been the initiator and founder of a non-profit foundation. The governor of her state has positioned her on a variety of state and community boards and she has been voted by numerous organizations as "the most outstanding women to..." She has all the right accoutrements: an office in the center of downtown, a stylish car, a car phone, a personal shopper, a hair designer, a therapist, and membership in the most prestigious professional clubs. In our converestion, I sensed she was covering up something. When I asked her, "What was life like as a child?" She said, "difficult." Ann described her parent's relationship toward each other as very cold and rigid. There was much tension because her father was an alcoholic. When Ann was a child, though, she had warm memories of her father. There was a closeness and love between them that gradually changed as she grew into her teen age years. Emotionally Ann and her father made a deep connection during this time and then moved apart. Ann remembered her mother never being available for her. Ann could never remember a time when she and her mother had an intimate time together since her mother distanced herself from Ann by being ineffective (which Ann interpreted as weak), hostile, and angry. Ann recalled a time when she was young that she made a decision not to be like her mother. As a teenager she wanted to escape and run away from the whole situation. Today, her mother has also become an alcoholic, thus keeping Ann more separated and distant than ever from both mother and dad.

Ann was the special one to her parents for seven years, until her brother was born. Ann excelled at school but as her brother grew older, he was in conflict with the family and was constantly in some kind of trouble. By the time he reached his twenties, with all the childhood traumas and teenage rebellion, he landed in jail. Guiltily, Ann's parents paid the bond for his release, but after the trial and his prison sentence, they never visited him. Ann took on this responsibility to visit her brother.

A good student in school, Ann was also involved in many extracurricular activities. She attended college, owned her own business, was married, and then divorced. The marriage lasted only a few years. She experienced difficulty in the marriage when her earning power exceeded that of her husband. His complaint was that she spent too much time with work and community activities, and little time with him. Basically, Ann easily aligns with the masculine qualities of being powerful, confident, and productive. She struggles with expressing such feminine qualities as being intuitive, expressing feelings, being sensitive, and allowing softness. She is aware that these feminine characteristics are difficult to express publicly so she has actively worked with a therapist to integrate some of them into her life.

Ann has had this insatiable masculine push of working hard because, as she shared, "I was the one chosen to uphold the family image because it was lost with my father's alcoholism and my brother's criminal record. I felt I was being told to be the one to win back the respect for our family." Ann has a strong Professional Pattern which is driven by her family's needs. This drive intensifies the constant need to be accepted and to be approved by the male society. Her high achievement skills also keep her on this treadmill. Ann chose to move away from her mother as a feminine model early in her life when there was a wide gap and lack of bonding with her. Men in the community have become her models.

Her Sensual Pattern cries out for expression because it is also at the core of her feminine energy, and it has long been neglected. The Professional Pattern has so overpowered her that it is only at night when she goes home alone to her apartment that she is aware of the feelings of loneliness. She pacifies this woundedness by being the heartful listener to many of her prominent male, married colleagues. She is always number two but never makes it to the number one position and thus goes home again, alone. Her Achilles heel is that she struggles whether to allow herself to let go to a deeper place inside, and to get in touch with the power of the Transition Pattern energy. There is a deep fear of finding the feminine core of her self. As she begins to contact her feminine core, she is reminded that to be feminine is to be weak, flaky, and unavailable, like her mother. She has remained unavailable to her own feminine just as her mother has remained unavailable to her.

Even though she has been in therapy for years, to allow herself to go blindly into this dark part of herself is difficult. Because reaching down into one's soul requires guidance, a female coach, a spiritual guide, or a therapist who can facilitate the process of going within and finding one's feminine core is needed. A male therapist, guide, or coach generally follows a different path, and has a fundamentally different psychological process for encountering the darkness within. It is difficult for a man to guide a woman on her path when she is willing to go through the death/rebirth process. Ann longs for a male companion. She wants a man that she can't rule over, or that she doesn't need to take care of emotionally, intellectually, or financially. She wants a relationship of heart and reciprocity.

Ann is a good example of a woman who is living the of Man-Made Woman Era. She has lived a male-programmed life, covering up her inner core as a woman. She learned early not to have any awareness of her own cadence as she marched to her family's dysfunction. She become overly-accountable and took on the job of redeeming the family name. The strong clue that Ann is beginning to move into the Emerging Woman Era was her high score on the Integrated Developmental Stage. This indicated that she is looking at herself from a different aspect and is beginning to see that the inner world of the feminine is also a missing link to fulfilling the black hole of her loneliness. Ann is beginning to learn that outer success is superficial and is not lasting. The exciting thing about Ann is that she is working hard at touching the power of her inner feminine, and she is setting the stage for the Emerging women to blossom within her.

At age 39, Ann's health was fairly good; she indicated no major illnesses. I have found, though, with most strong Professional Patterned women, that they have constant gastrointestinal problems, including upset stomach, constipation, hypoglycemia and headaches. Generally, they are allergic to different types of foods and the toxicity in the environment.

LESLIE

AGE: 55
CAREER: Volunteer, student, health professional
ERA: Passive Woman
PRIMARY PATTERN: Professional
SECONDARY PATTERN: Sensual/Outdoors
DEVELOPMENTAL STAGES: Integrator/Survivor
MEDICAL PROBLEMS: Back surgery, CFIDS, Hypothyroidism

Leslie's father died when she was four years old. Life was a struggle. When she was eight years old her mother remarried. Now life took on a whole new hue; it was wonderful until her step-father died three years later. She had fond memories of her step-father and she idolized him. She holds memories of spending lots of time with him until his death.

Leslie's mother became a survivor after living through the death and grief of two husbands, during the time of the 1929 depression. She had a teaching credential so she was able to find work. Leslie learned very early in her life the art of persistence, endurance, and responsibility. She started working at the age of 10, taking on the work role of her father. She worked in a doctor's office. The doctor, observing her drive and need to achieve, was a pivotal influence in Leslie's life. He was so impressed by her academic abilities and by her determination and earnestness that he gave her money to go to nursing school. She entered nursing school when 17 years old.

Leslie completed her training and was married at 21. Her husband was also a high-driving, achievement-oriented type man. While her children were young, she was director of a school of nursing. She wore many hats as a wife, mother, and a professional. Eventually, it got to be too much so she decided to leave her work and stay home. This was a trying time for Leslie because she loved working, and she had an intense need to be out in the world. She told me sadly, "I felt like I had retired to become a corporate wife and mother." When her girls were teenagers, she did contract work at a convalescent home, and while lifting a terminally ill patient, she broke her back.

After a long recovery from back surgery, Leslie wanted to extend herself into the world once again. She first volunteered in the community; she particularly enjoyed volunteering at the high school her children attended. She got involved in the counseling program and loved it. Currently, she is in the last year of her PhD program in counseling psychology.

After reflecting on her own story she said, *"I wished I was ten years younger. I felt my children took up so much of my time because I have such a strong desire to work and achieve."* Her frustration came from playing the passive woman roles but in her heart wanting to be in the man-made women arena. Maybe the pull between these two life styles created her subsequent illnesses.

Here is a woman with a strong internal Professional pattern but who has put her desires on the back burner for her professional man and her children. Her Sensual Pattern comes out with her husband. She says, "I am a different woman when I am with him. I act the sensual part, choosing feminine clothes, not being assertive, using my intuition, and being soft." She also shared, "But then I really feel powerless." It was hard for her to stay in touch with her sensual pattern. I found this pattern not as strong in her because the strong career pull influences her more to her masculine side. The Outdoors Pattern, with its intense push to keep physically active, has also been sabotaged from time to time by such traumas as the injury and back surgery. But her basic message to herself is: the "show must go on." She keeps incredibly busy.

Currently Leslie has immune and autoimmune problems. She has hypothyroidism as well as CFIDS. She spends most of her time in bed. She said, *"I am frustrated with my life. What I wanted to do was to feel more powerful but what I feel is so unfinished. It has cost me a lot to keep trying to achieve more and do more. I really do not know how to play. The work ethic instilled in my youth is so strong that it overpowers play time."* She does not have time to take personal care of herself; when she is competing with men in the work world, she becomes hardened and over-involved in tasks, objectives, and goals. With her illness, however, she has had to be quiet. As I discovered, this is one of the ways the body is trying to get her back in balance. Leslie's high achievement goals in a male-oriented world and her intense struggle to get there tends to keep her inner feminine energy from being expressed. The body defending itself against who she truly is places her high on the list for immune disease problems. In her childhood she learned the Survivor Developmental stage of the feminine and thrives on responsibility. Due to her lifestyle and illness, she has developed traits from the Integrator Developmental stage and has stopped most activities in order to take time to heal childhood wounds and balance her life.

The Sensual Woman Pattern

MARIAN

AGE: 41
CAREER: Director position
ERA: Man-Made Woman
PRIMARY PATTERN: Sensual
SECONDARY PATTERN: Outdoors and Family
DEVELOPMENTAL FEMININE STAGE: Integrator/ Survivor
MEDICAL PROBLEMS: Fibroma of the uterus, hysterectomy

The description of the Sensual Woman's Pattern was stated clearly by Marian when she said, "Men are a vehicle to get me to where I want to be in the world. I don't feel that I am good enough to compete on a man's terms; I am angry about it and alienated most of the time. But no matter what I put up with, it will get me to where I am going." Reflecting on her statement helps me understand why many of the women I've met have The Sensual Pattern as one of the top three patterns in their assessment profile. Marian has a childhood story that illustrates how The Sensual Woman Pattern was developed and how this pattern's charm assisted her to make it through an unfortunate beginning in her life.

For a woman to be married or to be with a man gives her acceptance from society; she can say, "See, I am OK, I am good enough, I have a man." Being with a man, then, serves to protect a woman from society's basic unacceptability of females. But just underneath the skin of most women is this "not enough" pain disguised as sweetness, niceness, and compliance. This, then, covers up anger and frustration, often resulting in bitchiness and carrying a chip on the shoulder.

Marian's childhood was arduous. She lived on a farm with her parents who were poor. Her parents were divorced when she was a year old; she was unaware that her stepfather was not her biological father until she was 13 years old. Her Mother blurted it out one day when they were arguing. In the argument, Marian had sided with him and her mother said, "Why are you defending your father? He is not even your real father!" Marian was devastated at this news. She was also confused as to why she had supported her stepfather because he gave her nothing but grief. Her stepfather had a drinking problem and was later diagnosed a schizophrenic. He abused her physically when he beat her with a belt buckle and sexually when he would come naked into her room at night. He also forced her to kiss him on the lips, when she wanted to get permission to go out on dates. Because of the stepfather's mental illness, her mother would not stand up for her children. Her mother, being uneducated, and with little chance for decent work, feared the worst if he left; she believed she could not financially take care of her family.

Marian became the surrogate mother and wife since she was the oldest of four children; her mother was also severely depressed. At times she felt honest love from her stepfather, but those times were few and far between. With the problems and responsibilities at home, it was hard for her to be a student, as well as mother and wife. Her only joy and favorite subject in school was art. At 16 years , she ran away from home and became a ward of the court. She was taken in by a professional woman and man who had no children. Marian was in heaven. There was no more abuse from her stepfather and she was given love and attention. From this couple she learned the social graces, learned about professional life, and about another life style.

While still a ward of the court, she married her high school sweetheart immediately after graduating from high school so she would not have to move back home. Soon after marrying, Marian discovered her husband was an alcoholic, and when he was drunk he would beat her. Working and caring for two small children, she could not continue holding the relationship together, so she asked for a divorce. This so angered her husband that he took a kitchen butcher knife and tried to kill himself by stabbing himself in the chest. Amazingly enough, she did not buy into this suicide attempt and he left the house alone to get help. Later, Marian heard his girlfriend, with whom he was secretly having an affair, assisted him in getting emergency care. She did not question the urgency of getting a divorce.

To get back on her feet and to support her family, Marian got a job in a bakery. There she tried to learn more skills in order to earn more; she wanted to move out of her poverty level existence. When the men took their coffee breaks, or vacations, she asked to learn how to operate the baking machines so she could fill any vacancy. All these positions were held by men so when she took over the baking machines it was quite an accomplishment. Within a few years, Marian remarried primarily to ensure that her children would have stability and financial support.

Her next step in moving out of the low economic lifestyle, was to become an entry-level secretary. But she always kept her eyes on the next advancing step. This next step came again by observing and helping out those women in the administrative assistant positions. When an opportunity opened, Marian applied for and became assistant to the president. With no formal college degree, she is now director of a department in a major corporation and earns over $100,000 a year.

Since Marian lacked the early model and drive of the high achievement Professional Pattern, how did she make it in the business world? Marian adapted the Sensual Pattern that runs on a different energy for success. Her success is in direct relationship with the success of the man with whom she is associated. In her steps out of poverty she connected with males by listening to their problems and becoming their intimate companion, whether sexual or verbal. She learned to be the "other woman" early, as a child, and this has been her primary survival mechanism. Being the "other woman" helped her to move from one position to another, up the economic ladder. Marian created her success without a college degree, through a strong fortitude to survive. She did it with her ability to connect and relate well with men.

Her Outdoors Pattern is the active energy that will keep Marian physically moving no matter what happens to her. She always kept her feet on the ground actively pursuing every possibility. Marian wasn't an idealist or a dreamer. Because nature sings inside of her, driving extra hours to live near the ocean is a must for her; she wants the out of doors nearby. On her off hours she works out with aerobic dancing, walking, quilting, and playing baseball. Her Family Pattern is quite typical in that she takes care of everyone and seeks to nurture them. It isn't a surprise to find many Family Pattern women working in restaurants or bakeries. Marrying for security to assure her children are cared for is more important than being in love. This is a typical Family Pattern. Her ability to problem solve and handle all kinds of chaotic crises is the Family Pattern's dream come true. Because of this characteristic love of solving problems, Marian has been an asset in the corporate setting. People are taken by her nurturance, and by her willingness to reach out, and give time and energy to them. How does she nurture herself? That is the irony of the Family Pattern. Recently Marian had an emergency hysterectomy, with ovarian fibroids almost closing off her intestines. This was a clear feminine call from the body to go inside and be touched, listened to, and held.

I wondered if Marian's illness had anything to do with her struggle of pretending that she is the Passive Woman, a servant to men, but in reality entrenched in the Man-Made Woman's whirl. She is a very strong woman, but needs to learn more about the feminine traits of intuition and personal rhythms which are developed in the Survivor stage of life. Marian became stuck, as most women leaders have, in the patterns for survival learned in childhood. Women like this need to be more conscious of their inner natural rhythms, insights, and intuitions. My fear for women like Marian who are successful in the man's world, is that they may never recapture their feminine strengths, feminine timing and inner knowing. Making it financially is no longer the issue, but the pattern and drive still tends to keep her off balance.

From their difficult childhoods, Ann and Marian have been driven to gain respect for themselves. I wondered, then, if we as women have been so diminished that we haven't enough self esteem we need to continually use men to gain our worth in this society.

VIRGINIA

AGE: 41
CAREER: Director position, Private Corporation
ERA: Man-Made

PRIMARY PATTERN: Sensual
SECONDARY PATTERNS: Family/Professional/Community/Transition/Outdoors.
DEVELOPMENTAL FEMININE STAGE: Fighter/Survivor
MEDICAL PROBLEMS: None Given

Virginia was the only woman I assessed who exhibited all feminine patterns in almost equal strength across the board. She was the oldest of three children and was the "good girl," helping to make life easier for her parents. Her mother was sick all the time, being a hypochondriac. Virginia took over being surrogate mother and wife, leaving the door open to being a father's daughter — living up to and nurturing what he wanted her to achieve. He encouraged Virginia to be an athlete. Although she tried, she was not as coordinated physically as her peers and she failed to meet her father's expectations. Even today she still tries, however, by getting out and walking some fourteen miles a week.

As a child she succeeded in school, developing her confidence and connecting her intelligence with Dad, and, thus, ultimately making him happy. Virginia's grandfather taught her unconditional love, integrating the Sensual Pattern of innocence, vulnerability, and intimacy. This becomes important for her working in the corporate world today. She had a grandmother who was the teacher and the nurturer, she was Virginia's model of the Family Woman Pattern. Virginia affectionately recalls those wonderful smells of homemade bread coming from her grandmother's kitchen.

As is often the case with such a strong woman, Virginia married a weaker man. Finally tired of the imbalance of her strength to his weakness along with his drinking and affairs, she divorced him. After that relationship ended, Virginia married her boss, a professional man. He became her mentor, and taught her how to apply her intellectual skills in the male business world. She was such a good student that she learned quickly and moved into the Professional Pattern of high achievement. She is currently in the directorship of a large corporation and is the first woman to hold such a position in the company. She is in line for a vice president position, but is experiencing the glass ceiling. She has looked for outer guidance concerning how to break through, but is now looking for inner guidance as she moves into the Transition Pattern.

What has happened to her Sensual Pattern with her husband as her Professional Pattern has grown? There is a level of her competence that has intimidated him. This is a challenge for the relationship to grow in different kinds of ways. Virginia's drive to experience her inner world often creates a gap between the two of them.

The Community Pattern mode is being developed as she becomes more and more involved in elected professional associations. Her sense of power, influence, strength, and confidence is rising as she excels in the community. As she excels more and more, Virginia feels more powerful, more the Warrior and Fighter stage, and believes she can be a positive influence in many situations. As she develops into all the patterns at once she is dynamic, loving, and powerful. This woman is a professional with heartful interest in taking care of others within the community. She is searching for more knowledge about herself and is trying to live a principle-centered life from the inside out. Since the ideal life was not what she experienced during childhood, there is a constant struggle to make up for what happened to her at the early Survivor Developmental Stage. She drives herself by putting great emphasis on the care of the family. The danger for a woman like Virginia is not learning her own biological, emotional, and mental, rhythms and not listening intuitively to her own needs. By focusing back into the window of her life where she took on more than was needed as a young girl, she gained her strength and insight to restructure the patterns learned at that time. Doing this will prepare her for the next stage, that of the Integrator Crone.

JEAN

AGE: 50
CAREER: CEO of her own company
ERA: Man-Made
PRIMARY FEMININE PATTERNS: Sensual
SECONDARY FEMININE PATTERNS: Professional/ Community
DEVELOPMENTAL STAGES: Idealizer/Fighter
MEDICAL PROBLEMS: None Given

At the end of World War II in Greece, Jean's mother was pregnant with her as her family escaped to Italy, England, and finally, to the United States. This tragedy was the motivating force that created a close-knit family. Jean was nurtured, loved, and given as much as possible in her childhood, even though life was unstable. She said, "I really didn't understand my mother until I was in my 30s and had children of my own." As a child she spoke mainly Greek; she couldn't speak English very well and she had a different accent from the rest of her school mates. Being different, she was discriminated against and ostracized by her peers. Thus, she spent most of her time with her family, even going to adult parties with parents. As a result she felt older than her classmates. It wasn't until her college years that she finally had some friends of her own age.

She learned quite early to be the Fighter, not only from

her experience at school, but also she was trained by her father, a strict disciplinarian. Although he imposed distance between them, she nonetheless idolized him. He admitted he was disappointed at not having a boy; Jean said, "I was the son my father wanted to have." Even so, he was traditional in the way he raised his girls. For example, girls didn't climb trees or stay out late at night. He also taught her as he would have a son, to have ambitious, driving, charging, competitive energy. She said, "I was trained to be both a good male and a pretty good female. I have the female personality but I also have more male personality than most men." Her father trained her into two strong patterns, the Sensual and the Professional Patterns.

He would instruct her in ways to be competitive; even at the dinner table there was usually competitive verbal dialogue to keep her on her toes. Jean respected her father and would go to him to help solve her problems, thus incorporating more of his values and thinking processes into her own style. Using him as her model, she, too, became headstrong; she wanted to be like him to prove to him that she was the best. He said to her, "Act like a man in these ways and look like a women in these ways." Of all the women I met in my research of women in leadership, Jean was the only women who was purposely trained by her father to live and work in a man's world.

For the first time in her life, however, she rebelled against her father in order to get away from his dominating influence. She consciously married a man her father's opposite and she became like her father. Jean adopted the Professional Pattern; she was the competitive, hard-driving Man-Made Woman and, he, the husband, played the soft, tender, right-brained woman role. Of course, this didn't work for long, but long enough to produce two

children. Jean's second husband is as strong and as powerful as she and there is more of a balance. Actually, she is
balancing the Sensual and Professional patterns just as
her father instructed her to do. She uses her wardrobe as
the way to act out the Sensual Pattern and has learned
also to be aggressive, pushy, and competitive as a she
adopts the male role — she has combined the two patterns.
The Community Pattern is also surfacing in Jean's life.
The last time I spoke to her, she had been elected to the
board of a major university and had influenced the hiring
of a new president of the university. She is starting plans
to create, and be the driving force for, a business school
located in Europe.

As for her physical health, Jean was one of the most
healthy women I met. She indicated that she has just
missed a handful of days of work in her entire career; she
works out every morning at a gym, arising by 5:00 a.m. She
focuses her attention on her body and stays healthy. She
has also thought out her priorities concerning what she
enjoys doing and what she doesn't enjoy doing; thus, many
of her needs are taken care of by others such as house-
keeper, cook, gardener, and personal shopper. Conse-
quently, she can totally concentrate on herself and on her
business.

The Transitional Woman Pattern
I was shocked to encounter so many Transitional Patterns in women in the research project. Although most of
these women worked in the healing arts, others worked in
the educational and business sector. I was pleased to find
so many searching women willing to risk going into the
dark hole of their subconscious selves. Digging deep within
is the prerequisite of shifting into The Emerging Woman
Era. Without doing the intense personal work, I believe
that it will be impossible for women to move away from the

role of always being number two in our society. Women will continue to repeat the same roles and patterns in the male-dominant society that they have known for centuries. What will we then be leaving for our children and for our children's children? I was heartened, actually ecstatic, with these results. The following women bore the markings of engaging in the Transition Pattern.

ANGIE

AGE: 53
PROFESSION: University professor
ERA: Passive
PATTERNS: Transition/Man-Made
SECONDARY PATTERNS: Sensual and Soul
DEVELOPMENTAL STATES: Explorer/Fighter
MEDICAL PROBLEMS: Rheumatoid arthritis, hypothyroid, food allergies

Angie was a tomboy, and loved her solitude. Her external world was uneventful which created much internal pain for her. She said it was devoid of nurturing because she was not stimulated or touched very much by her mother. Actually, Angie didn't talk until she was about 6 years old. She never remembered her mother holding her; in fact, she remembers that her mother put her in the playpen one day, on the porch, and forgot her out there. When it got dark, and her father came home from work, he found Angie and brought her into the house.

Angie's mother was very directive but also very much under the control of her own parents until they passed away. When Angie's grandparents died, Angie's mother finally married her father. She remembered her mother as extremely emotional, reacting to behaviors and situations with screaming temper tantrums, she was unable to forgive. She encouraged Angie to adopt a failing attitude. Her mother would say, "Angie, you are too sensitive, you will never make it in the world." Angie was taught nothing about money, sex, nor given any cooking skills. The only encouragement offered by her mother was to give Angie courage to go to college. Angie believes now, as an adult, that her mother was angry at her. Her Mother would say to Angie, "You stole my husband from me." The night Angie's father died, her mother was drunk and told Angie awful things about her father and admitted that she didn't know how to be a mother.

Angie's father, on the other hand, was nurturing; they went places together, he talked with her on many different subjects, and she loved hearing him tell stories about his life. She remembered him as a kind and good person. Dad was important to her because he helped her understand her female nature and also pointed out to Angie her intuitive ability. He encouraged her to understand and develop this ability. The most hurtful thing her father said to her happened when Angie and her mother were arguing one time. Her father said, "If this fighting continues, I am going to have to take the side of your mother, I will not take your side." Angie had felt she had an unbreakable bond with her father but, in the end, he sided with her mother. Angie's story exemplifies the Sensual Pattern of being number two and never making it to number one. Her deep feelings of inappropriate love of her father kept her from marrying for the rest of her life.

As a child she had polio which left her health weakened. Also being dyslexic created reading problems in school but she was helped while attending a Catholic school, with the discipline and extra attention. Angie had always gravitated toward crafts and artistic projects and she became an occupational therapist. She was kicked out of college because of bad grades and absences due to an illness, mononucleosis. Once out of college Angie continued her search to connect to others, reaching for that missing bond between her mother and herself; she eventually gravitated toward a hippie lifestyle and lived in a commune.

The Transitional Pattern of searching led Angie to meeting a male professor, an older man who acted as her mentor and her lover. He guided her through a Master's Degree, Ph.D. in psychology, and in getting her marriage, child, and family license. She researched and wrote her dissertation on a woman's journey into the dark night of the soul. This subject is of strong interest to the Transitional Pattern. For a time Angie and her mentor lived together but, true to the Sensual Pattern, she chose a married man who eventually returned to his wife. Again and again the cycle replayed and, later, Angie became ill with ovarian cancer and had to have a hysterectomy. Most of her intimate relations with men ended with her being left alone, the man would return to his wife or to another woman.

Although Angie became the dean of a university and fit into the Man-Made Era, when the restructuring of the department and conflict with her woman superior occurred, the stress was too much for her. Her sensitive tender heart, strong ideals, and values kept her from changing to the new direction the system was heading. Angie transferred the unresolved anger with her mother onto her female boss. As a result, at 49 years of age, Angie developed swollen joints and excruciating pain, a condition which resembled rheumatoid arthritis. She became crippled. This disease evolved into painful immobility; eventually, Angie had to leave her work and could do nothing but sit day after day in a chair in front of the television set. Within five years, being in constant pain and with many difficulties living alone and growing weaker, Angie died.

The Transition Pattern had been strong in Angie, however, as this is what her father had taught to her. He had said, *"Follow your intuition and have a religion, you can do anything you want to do."* He also was her mate as a child and imagined lover; she had a strong connection with him, so much so that she was never able to be with another man permanently. She longed for a relationship with a man who would not leave her for another woman.

The Soul Pattern started out early for Angie, when she failed to speak until 6 years of age. Because of not talking, she developed a strong inner world. And then, during her illness, and at the end of her life, she was also isolated and very much inside herself. She allowed herself to sink deeply into the darkness, into the abyss of her soul, and she elected not to return to life.

Angie needed the Fighter Development Stages to bring the feminine into her life. Angie needed to be more of her own authority and leader, thus removing her emotional dependence from her father. Even though her father was dead, there was still a dream, a fantasy, of waiting to be taken care of by a man like dad. Angie was physically overtaken by the emotional upheaval relating to the university departmental conflict; this experience left her incapable of engaging in the battle.

Women who have difficulty or chose not to move into the Man-Made Woman Era generally do not have the foundation gained from the Fighter Developmental Stage. Taking the upper hand and fighting the disease was what Angie needed to learn from the Fighter Stage. As a child, Angie's familiar response was to run to her father or escape inside herself. This is the Passive Woman's game plan. Angie needed strength from her feminine warrior; this would have changed her life.

She was strong tomboy and she tried to be like her brother, because her mother had accepted him but had rejected her. As Angie's resistance to her mother grew stronger, transitioning into womanhood to be like mother was difficult. And, Angie never really had a lasting relationship with a man other than her father. In the Feminine Development stage of Perfecter, this part of Angie's feminine was not developed. It would have been helpful if Angie had been able to go back, reexamine, and heal the pain with the disconnection to that stage of feminine development; the feminine could have emerged and may have brought balance to her life. Probably the key factor in the lives of most therapists is that they will tend to be high in the feminine Explorer Developmental Stage. Angie searched for an answer to her pain, and to understanding the hate for her mother, until she could search no further — she then died. Healing the thoughts focused on hating the feminine in oneself can heal the place in the body where the hateful, negative thoughts have been stored. Rheumatoid arthritis is an autoimmune disease that reflects self-attack, particularly woman hating herself as a female. Angie was unable to forgive her mother for rejecting and abandoning her as a child — Angie could no longer bear the notion of being like this mother, a woman incapable of nurturing her own child.

ELLEN

AGE: 49
CAREER: Art therapy
ERA: Passive
PRIMARY PATTERN: Transition
SECONDARY PATTERN: Outdoors/Professional
DEVELOPMENTAL FEMININE STAGES: Explorer/
  Survivor
MEDICAL PROBLEMS: Food and environmental allergies, candida, hypothyroidism

Ellen was the only child in an affluent family from the South. Her family moved seven times in thirteen years because her father's business was building homes, living in them for a time, and then selling them for investment purposes. Ellen loved her father, who was rarely at home because he worked so much, but he retired at forty-five years of age. She remembered times when she hid in the back seat of her father's truck just to be with him. He would find her and take her back home. She longed to be with him because she was terrified of her mother. Ellen's mother would yell at her in front of her friends, and was also rude and cold toward her. Ellen recalled a time when her father had broken a plate; her Mother severely blamed and punished her for this action. Not until dad arrived home did the truth emerge, but Ellen never received an apology from her mother. Her parents eventually divorced.

Ellen was shy, introverted, and non-verbal. Like Angie, Ellen spent time alone. She found solace with her horses, in the outdoors, and with her guitar and her books. School was a frightening experience for Ellen; it wasn't until the fourth grade, in an Episcopal school structure, and in a caring relationship with these teachers, that she began to excel differently. Ellen said, "I never memorized facts. I would always see them in patterns to remember them." Her mother loved art, saw artist possibilities in Ellen, and forced this art interest onto Ellen, hoping that Ellen would become what she herself was unable to attain. Ellen became driven by her mother's ambition, caught between her parents' power play. Her mother pushed her in one direction, out into the world, and her father pulled her back toward him. Both parents kept her tied to them in different ways. Her father's influence concerned money. Ellen said her father's philosophy was, "You need my money now, I don't want to wait to give it to you when I die. Don't worry, honey, I will support you so that you can be free, independent, and not have to be supported by a man." Her father's philosophy is that money brings one freedom and that is what he wants for Ellen. Rather than giving her independence, however, the parental ties strongly held Ellen; mother made decisions about her career and life work, while her father supervised how her money would be spent.

As an adult, then, Ellen had difficulty making decisions. Her mother directed her to go to art school even though Ellen's college vocational tests showed talents related to lab technician or librarian. Ellen also dated boys who would make all the decisions for her. As a young adult, she viewed herself as a sexually neutral person; her mother's lack of affection was coupled with repeated cautions about the fear and intrusion of sex and sexual diseases. Ellen lacked the permission she needed from her mother to be truly female. At thirty-three she changed her name from Lynn to Ellen, an overt symbol that she wanted a new identity, she wanted to be her own person. Ellen worked as an art designer and, as she began to regain her personal power and feel stronger, she went back to school and enrolled in an art therapy program. She wanted to creatively use her talent in art as a kind of therapy, to better understand herself.

Currently, Ellen is designing and selling homes similar to her dad. She has experienced a lesbian relationship and, now, is in an intimate relationship with a man. Ellen says, "The relationship with my own gender brought me nurturing and companionship with a women that I had never known; this also strengthened my values and my sense of personal empowerment. I am able to stand up for myself, honoring both myself and others. Since in a relationship with a man, tenderness has come back into my life — sweetness, and love. I am more free with myself than I have ever been."

As Ellen continues to unravel and cut the ties that have so tightly bound her to her mother she is moving through the Passive Woman Era. And her struggle is to also cut the ties with father and to be financially independent. What would happen if she broke free and become her own person? There would be a mutation of resourcefulness, strength, growing up, and independence that would change Ellen's life and connect her with a new model, that of the new Emerging Woman. To make this transformation, however, she must delve into feminine qualities that were not developed in the Survivor Stage, those of her own inner rhythms, timing, and risk. She has experienced the Explorer Development Stage, traveling to many cultures and traveling deep into her self. This is part of Ellen's feminine that has been raised to a conscious level, and is opening her independence. She is actively working on winning this battle; thus, her Transition Pattern matches the development of the feminine in the search for her true, and complete, feminine self. The Professional Pattern is represented by keeping closely aligned in similar business ventures to her father's. There is also a need to be close to both the earth and to the plant life. Ellen is currently living on ten acres in the country. Her gift is also working with communities of women to explore women's history and to integrate women's rituals into our lives. This is a strong indication of the Outdoor Pattern flourishing in Ellen's life.

The Outdoors Woman Pattern

I wondered how an Outdoors Pattern would influence women working in an office setting — could they manage indoors? The women I interviewed tended to choose positions and lifework that kept them on the go and not behind a desk. For example, the Outdoor Pattern women I talked with held political positions and were strong proponents of women's rights and women's well being. I also spoke with women who focused on women's health issues —for example, a physician whose speciality was Obstetrics and Gynecology. Thus, these women were leaders in a different way from the other patterns. They were forced into the male-dominant world by strong mothers. These daughters became fiercely independent and outspoken concerning what they believed, for themselves and for others. Here are two examples:

TERRY

AGE: 39
CAREER: Attorney
ERA: Man-Made
PRIMARY PATTERN: Outdoors
SECONDARY PATTERN: Professional/Sensual
DEVELOPMENTAL STAGES: Fighter/Survivor
MEDICAL PROBLEMS: Overweight

Terry was born into an academic family, with both parents engaged in teaching and research. Terry was a shy, skinny, insecure tomboy, and a bit rebellious. In the eighth grade, when she turned thirteen years old, she started gaining weight; this weight has stayed with her most of her life. Terry's mother was absorbed in her own work; she was always the tough, cool, judgmental teacher. Her father was buried in his books, occasionally would surface but not for long. He was much more human with his humor and warmth and was an eccentric, stubborn individual. Terry's older brother was her friend and companion; he offered her some advice, "Whatever you do, Terry, don't live at home after you finish high school." She did not heed this advice.

Terry tried to follow her brother's footsteps however — he was a good student and went to the University Lab School. For the most part, school did not occupy her imagination, and, in fact, she had anxiety about it. She didn't enjoy school work but she excelled in basketball, track, and swimming. Although Terry lived at home while she went to college, she survived living through the bitter conflict of her parent's deteriorating marriage. Years later, her parents divorced after being together forty-three years. Terry's somewhat sheltered existence living at home may have brought on an untimely pregnancy, marriage, and caused her not to finish college.

Terry's marriage lasted ten years, then ended in divorce. She went back to school, finished her degree, and also earned a law degree. Terry's, son, at seventeen years, had a mental breakdown and was diagnosed manic depressive. Although he lives on his own, her son's pain is a major concern. Terry then remarried, but her new husband suffered a stroke which will confine him to a wheelchair for the rest of his life. Terry's comment about her life situation: "I am learning to depend on my own self; and to think things through, now. My current husband is a burden but my first husband held my happiness back, too. When I enter my house after work, my mother, my husband and my dog all look at me longingly as if I am supposed to give them life."

Terry is living the life of the Man-Made Woman Era; she has plunged into the achievement-oriented male dominant world with all that goes along with it. Terry as the Outdoor Woman Pattern, is constantly on the go. Her comment to me was, "I need more leisure time for my self." Terry was the only woman I interviewed who saw no difference between the feminine and the masculine qualities. She said, "My male friends are just like my female friends in terms of the masculine and feminine qualities, I see no difference." This kind of comment is typical of the Outdoors Pattern in that the male companions are just as close as their women friends. Terry doesn't need to live in the country. She said she would be happy if she could be mowing her lawn rather than cooped up in an office. The Professional Pattern is also strong from her childhood; from the modeling by both parents. Terry followed their lead into an academic and professional life. My concern is that Terry's primary pattern may be squeezed out by the Professional Pattern. The Sensual Pattern of heartful connection to men is still alive; she is a good listener and friend to men but she said, "If it wasn't for the prevalence of sexual diseases I would probably still be single; I love being independent with many partners and I still desire the sexy fun."

Terry is immersed in the Survivor Developmental Stage as she struggles with being responsible for many people in her world. She may be taking so much responsibility for others that she neglects herself. The Explorer Developmental Stage has not had a chance to blossom in Terry to bring forward the inner feminine's expression. Having a family at such a young age, then putting herself through school, and, now, taking on the total responsibility for family does not leave time or impetus to open the doors for inner exploration. Terry learned, in the Development Stage of the Fighter, that she needed to be responsible for her ill son and find a way of taking care of him as well as herself. Returning to school and, now, beginning to manage others is bringing forward in Terry the feminine mode of leadership and community development. When she is able to proceed in this direction, Terry will begin to carry the energy of the Emerging Woman. When she chooses this path, however, it must be through both the body and the intellect.

DENISE

AGE: 49
CAREER: Judge
ERA: Man-Made
PRIMARY PATTERN: Outdoors
SECONDARY: Sensual/Community
DEVELOPMENTAL STAGES: Fighter/Survivor
MEDICAL PROBLEMS: Polio

Denise's childhood was a struggle for her independence from her overpowering mother. Even though her mother was quiet and well educated, she was strong-willed, ambitious, and dominating. As the oldest child, Denise received love and support from her family but there was always the conflict between being independent or being ruled by her mother. As a child, Denise had contracted polio which accounted for her need to be dependent and cared for by her mother. Her father was a civil engineer, who was supportive, humorous, outgoing, and affable. Denise was not close to either of her parents.

School was not easy for Denise and she wasn't a great student, but she committed to putting herself through college. After graduating from college, she married and had two children. Staying at home with the children and doing housework was increasingly boring to Denise; she sought out ways to bring some meaning into her life. The League of Women Voters introduced her to the women's movement in 1960 and she became intensely involved with the National Organization for Women (NOW), working on equal rights for women. So convinced was Denise that she wanted to facilitate and be more influential in changing the laws and making social policy, that she decided to enter law school. Her goal was to be a policy-maker but she lacked confidence to speak in front of crowds. Denise first worked in political caucus organizations, and with domestic violence issues. She became a judge for Native Americans and, then, acted as a legal court advocate to help women.

Denise worked for ten years to build her confidence and when she took the risk to run for an office, she was elected. Denise said, "I like to make changes; the system is not set up for women but I have been successful in politics because I have played their (men's) system. Although I have had to become another man, I hope I have brought things to the table that wouldn't have come from a man's perspective. It is hard to assess how much I have changed; I am headstrong and I have championed issues for woman that men have not. I can be very threatening and have made my male colleagues uncomfortable because I speak directly when I have been backlashed by men."

Denise's comment impressed me as being viable for one working from the Man-Made Woman Era. Once Denise was attending a night meeting with her colleagues. In the meeting she continued to have conflict with one of the male attenders. After the meeting, she went to her office, put her head on her desk, and cried. After a good cry, she felt better and then went home. When she arrived at her office the next morning, on her desk was an unsigned memo which read, "Don't cry in your office." The norm of not showing emotions and feelings in the male-dominated work environment serve to continually hold back the feminine, when women must emulate men.

The Outdoor Pattern is Denise's predominant feminine pattern. Her pattern is marked with doing and being an out-front spokesperson for her community. Also an integral part of the Outdoors Pattern is her allegiance to women, and the importance to her of having positive relationships with women. Denise wanted me to share with readers her strong belief that women leaders must also have a community of women around them as friends. She said it was important because it is very lonely at the top. She went on to say that sometimes, on her way home from the office, she will stop at a woman friend's home, knock on the door and say, "Do you have a moment to talk? I am lonely, I need to talk."

The Sensual Pattern is exemplified in Denise's life by her awareness of how the sexual aspect of being a women affects men; she is concerned that it does not overpower them. As a public figure, she must be attentive to any behaviors that could be interpreted as using feminine wiles to manipulate decisions. She is concerned that the sensual part of her does not threaten either men or women and she is sensitive and open to talking and listening to others' feelings. The Community Pattern is very active with her intense desire to better the community; by being elected to public office, she has the power to identify problems and influence their solutions. Her concern about how she looks and appears to others is an important aspect of the Community Pattern.

Denise's Survivor Stage was overly-developed because she has become one of those women who takes on the responsibility for the entire world. She is somewhat aware of her life rhythms, however, and stops her busy pace to travel occasionally in order to rejuvenate herself physically and emotionally.

The goal of surfacing the nurturing feminine is not to wait until one needs to stop and rejuvenate, but rather to consciously allow the feminine to surface every moment of the day. Denise needs to uncover the feminine aspect from the Explorer Stage to bring to consciousness her strong inner mind power as a part of her driving force rather than her masculine outgoing external power. From Denise's story we can notice that she has developed her feminine from the Fighter Developmental Stage. Denise's desire for the good of women's lives and for her community's well being has encouraged her to fight for an opportunity to be in an influential position in order to make these things happen. She truly is an example of the feminine rising to the heights of the Fighter Stage.

The chart below gives an overview of The Feminine Model.

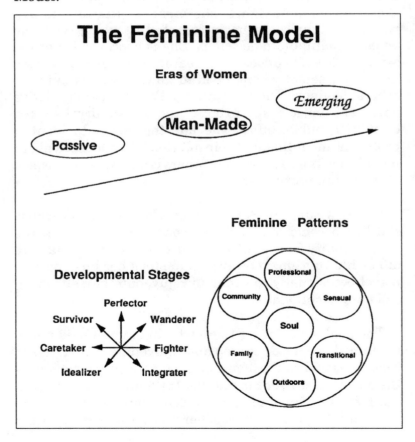

7. The Emerging Woman, who is she? Why is she important?

*Freedom is what you do with what's been
done to you.*

Jean-Paul Sartre

When Sleeping Beauty woke up she knew her life had changed. Unfortunately, it wasn't the prince's kiss that had awakened her. Rather than the prince, I believe an extraordinary experience changed her perception. When she awoke she felt differently, she thought differently, and she acted differently. What was this disruptive impact? Why did it affect her so deeply?

Many of us are Sleeping Beauties and I believe momentous life changes such as a decline in health, changes in the body, loss of significant relationships, loss of job positions, or, lack of professional advancements can trigger a substantial change and create insights in our fundamental belief system. Dramatic transformational encounters can plunge a woman deeply within herself. As Marion Woodman says, *"Transformation moves energy from the unconscious to the conscious."*[1] The Emerging Women is, like Sleeping Beauty, transformed and awakened into a new world.

But if women get stuck in the death stages and do not awaken they will die in their own spoiled debris or, like Sleeping Beauty, stay dead in their glass coffins. I believe this unconscious form of demise is encouraged in our culture. The tradition wields its insidious power, forces us to remain asleep, inhibiting our personal growth. Women must reach into the darkness and touch their abandoned soul, the container of their conscious feminine energy in order to survive and grow today. For centuries we have struggled against odds to be rescued and resurrected from our own darkness. And the conscious feminine has waited and waited like Sleeping Beauty for this reconnection. A woman who has touched this energy emerges genuine, real, and authentic. When the separated feminine is reconnected — to herself, a woman regains her own source of life and power.

The poet John Milton, describes Adam and Eve as *"He for God only, she for God in him."*[2] The conscious feminine, however, eliminates Adam as a mediator to her source of power. This elimination can be both frightening and challenging, to bring the feminine consciousness from the dark abyss of Inanna into the light. Women who remain within the darkness say, "Without a man I would not exist, so I will have to become just like a man in order to get my power." Women who choose to reconnect with the light of the conscious feminine say, "I want to be myself — and I choose to embrace and follow my own purpose and direction." This change in the focus of many women has resulted in a threat to the dominator society, and challenges its hard-won masculinity.

I changed after my mountain experience; but I had no idea there would be so many ramifications. To my surprise, it resulted in a change in my thinking process and the way I viewed the world. My home was uprooted and I journeyed, like Inanna, into my body. The mountain event was my first conscious meeting with the feminine energy. It was confusing, it felt romantic, and it didn't involve a man — it was self generated. It came from inside myself. Because of this, it touched a powerful creative resonance of the feminine in my body and I began to give birth to myself.

An unconscious part of me feared that if I had acted on this powerful energy, however, I would not be assured of staying safe and secure in the traditional masculine-based world. I did not know what to do without the authoritarian approval. As a result, I denied the activation of the feminine power, searched for more mountain experiences, got scared, put my life on hold, and whirled into dis-ease.

I had experienced the feminine energy but my body and my self esteem were not yet strong enough for it. I have learned that the feminine energy lives in physical matter, the body and nature. I have also learned that the container, the body, must be healthy and be consciously accepted by us in order for the unconscious feminine to be unveiled. I went through trials and tribulations to remove the veil — psychologically, physically, and spiritually. My professional, left-brained, masculine lifestyle taught me to think in my head and not to listen, or be aware of, my body. I needed to accept my body and become aware of how my body felt. I had knowledge of how it functioned but I had no conscious awareness or experience of the body's felt sense. My illness gave me the opportunity to open up the channels of awareness, and connect my body to myself — particularly in the way my body functioned and how I was to keep it healthy. Woodman describes the movement of this energy, *"Bringing the feminine component out of mystique and into consciousness is a healing process. . . Locating the disowned feminine in dreams and bringing it into realization, not through the intellect, but through the body, reestablishes harmony."*[3]

After I had compiled and studied the results of the women's research project, I noticed similar transitions reflected in some of the women I had interviewed. They also had experienced a forced radical shift, and many had cut old ties, breaking through to their core nature as a woman.

I knew some undercurrent movement was encouraging

women to change their inner and outer selves. These women connected to their inner feminine garden, through a body experience. I believe we get sick to learn that the body is the essential container of life, and through the healing process learn not to become handicapped or dependent on authority. The acceptance of my body and taking responsibility for it is a new perception. Just 100 years ago the law read, *"A woman's body belongs to her husband; she is in his custody, and he can enforce his right by a writ of habeas corpus."*[4] I had to learn to focus, concentrate, and listen to the needs of my body, regarding several factors: the type and amount of exercise, my dietary and sleep requirements, my personal energy patterns, and, my individual bodily rhythms. The willingness to learn is crucial for the *emergence of the conscious feminine.*

Marion Woodman presents the next step in our awakening when she suggests that the feminine, *"Allows the body to become a chalice for the reception of the spirit."*[5] I believe that a partnership system is paramount to the survival of the planet Earth and I believe the conscious feminine is the missing link in both men and women. If the Emerging Feminine is to be the holder of the masculine spirit energy, a woman must be an equal on both the outer and the inner levels of herself. The feminine must have a firm, established base for uniting with the masculine spirit. To be an equal with a man the feminine foundations must first be laid down internally. I was taught it was the other way around — that women were to know and connect with the masculine base first, and never truly know what her feminine life was really like.

As women wake up from years of internal, emotional, and spiritual imprisonment, they need models to follow. They need women who have emerged from the deep sleep and can act as mentors. When they hear other women's stories of significant shifts, and life changes, I hope they will feel inspired and also feel safe to allow the feminine to begin to emerge in themselves. It is through the education of women, by women, sharing with other women, that this awakening will grow, spread, and build a vortex of positive energy. This change will not be legislated; rather, it will happen by personal evolvement and personal empowerment.

While doing the research project, I met two women who had fallen into the deep death hole; connected with their feminine energy, and came back to life. The compassionate sharing of their stories put my own plight into perspective. Judy was one of these woman. She is a COO being groomed to be a CEO of a major national corporation. When I met her in her office, her appearance was of authoritarian strength, efficiency, and remoteness. These were the right male attributes. I immediately saw a softness in her eyes, however, and I heard a tenderness in her voice which I hadn't perceived in many professional women. I knew she had made a shift and I wondered if she would tell me about her experience.

Judy openly discussed her dysfunctional family back-ground. The eldest of three children, she became a surro-gate mother as early as six years old because her mother was emotionally and physically incompetent. She said she listened to her mother's problems, made family decisions, and went to the bank on the bus at six years old. Her alcoholic father was not home most of the time, but when he was at home, he was often argumentative. At times, he would push them around using his gun. Judy feared coming home from school even though she felt warmth from her father. This warmth from her father was one of her fondest childhood memories. She was not, however, supported by her family in her transition into womanhood. Judy's father made sexual putdowns about her physical changes, and physically wrestled with her, causing some physical injury.

At the age of 15, her home situation got so bad that she moved in with her grandmother. This move initiated her mother's decision to leave her father. I think Judy being the surrogate wife, together with her father's unconscious sexual advances, created a codependent relationship between Judy and her father. This encouraged the feminine Sensual Pattern to cast a shadow over her future male relationships. As she learned to compensate in school for the disruptions at home, she became an over-achiever, class officer, and athlete.

She followed her family's model and married an alcoholic man which resulted in years of struggle. Her marriage ended in her late thirties after she determined to change her environment and have a life for herself. Judy put herself though college and took a job in a large company as a trainer. Within 14 years she climbed to the top of the corporation and became Chief Operating Officer.

I have heard many stories of families that had forced women to be overly-responsible, and divorces that initiated independence, but I still questioned what had happened to Judy? She shared that, in her middle forties, as a single parent and while building her career, she received a telephone call informing her that her 17-year-old son had been killed in an automobile accident. Tears came to her eyes as she told me about his death. I knew this was the life event that changed her reality. This jolt disrupted her life and created an unimaginable loss which sent her spiraling downward into death. She said, "When you are turned inside out and your defenses are gone it is much easier to open up and start to become who you are because it is just too hard to keep the cover on any longer."

Judy plunged into the grieving and healing process, supported by her family and friends. Her basic feminine pattern is the athletic Outdoors Pattern and, innately, she chose a type of therapy called bioenergetics. This method utilizes the body as a resource and storehouse of personal memories. This therapy helped heal the pain from the death of her son and, subsequently, the childhood pain of her inner child. Upon Judy's spiral upward, and, with her mask removed she says, "I now do exactly what I want to do." She loves her work, often visits her children and grandchildren, exercises, enjoys bike trips, travels, and encourages people in her company to "do their work," which is what she calls their inner healing.

Now Judy is taking another plunge, or as she says, "I am taking the next step." She is about to break through the "glass ceiling." In a matter of months, her executive board will cast the deciding vote to make Judy their next CEO. "It is both "frightening and exciting," she says, "to be the first women CEO in this system which employees 82 per cent women." Judy also revealed that she is in an internal shift as well as being in her professional transition. Her metaphor is, "I am crossing a rushing current of water with one foot solidly resting on the next rock. The other foot has not yet lifted." She explained, "I have done the inner child work; now I am working with a dysfunctional-family counselor and I am confronting the issues around parenting. I have sat down with many friends and cleaned up conflicting issues. Many relationships have deepened and some have dropped away. To be successful in my next step I can't keep taking care of people."

In the three years since Judy took the COO position, employees have remarked about the changed company environment. People have said about her that she is too honest and too tough, but when reprimanded, they can feel that she cares, and they told her that in a crisis she has an incredible ability to focus. Judy has brought feminine principles into the company. One example is, after a routine employment opinion survey, she met in small groups with 1,860 employees to hear their opinions and establish a positive rapport. This is something no one at any level has ever initiated in the company. The results are that, at major decision-making meetings people feel they are heard, respected, and can openly share about their concerns.

"The leader of the future," Judy said, "is one who may have all the leadership skills in the world, but who won't be able to lead until they have done their inner work." With that thought in mind, she encouraged the officers in her company to go through a team building effort with two polarity therapists. Polarity therapy is another body therapy that encourages one to uncover inner memories that may hamper the health and well being of the individual.

In preparation for the executive board's vote, Judy's direct reports have evaluated her on 300 characteristics that can make or break her as the next CEO. The list included areas of competency and operational skills as well as relational and personal characteristics. On a scale of 1 to 5, her over-all score was 4.5. She was delighted with the results but the next hurdle is for the executive board to interview her on some of her weaker areas. What man would have to be put through such rigors to become a CEO?

I think the most important Emerging Woman statement Judy made was when asked what was driving her to take this position. She said, "It is not the money, although I want to be appropriately compensated; and I don't need to be the first women CEO in this system even though I have been a frontierswoman. The reason I want the position as CEO *is to see what I can achieve in creating an environment with the feminine principles.* I have seen what can be done in three years; I know it can work and be even more successful. The universe has chosen me to take this company through a time of significant transition. Will I take it through the change or will it have to be closed down? I don't yet know."

Whatever is the next step for Judy, this Emerging Women has already made great strides to establish within her body a strong inner feminine framework as her basic learning foundation. With the feminine qualities of personal integrity, honesty, and relational skills, she has integrated her outer expression of masculine skills to further her communication, logic, and organization skills. A personal partnership has been established within herself.

I met with another Emerging Woman, Erica, who was recovering from CFIDS. I was struck by her invigorated energy and depth. As she shared her story about strong professional parents, she talked lovingly of her dominant Middle-Eastern father who controlled her childhood by his eruptive anger and torrid passion. She spoke also of her northern European mother's intellectual, stoic strength. Erica knew her father loved her, and she loved to match him with her bubbly spirit and her outgoing personality. As a sensitive child, however, she took on her parents unexpressed emotional pain; as an adult she felt controlled and burdened by this responsibility.

Upon graduation, Erica taught high school and was awarded for teaching controversial subjects such as death and aging. Although she was close to her parents and it was hard to leave home, she moved across the country after being accepted into graduate school. It was then she met an extraordinary woman, a spiritual teacher who greatly influenced Erica's life. This woman was a compelling teacher. Erica was captivated by her and worked non-stop to become her right-hand person for ten years.

Erica related well with both men and women but remained more partial to women. Her female teacher strongly objected to this attraction and tried to "cure" Erica's homosexuality. Her teacher purported to be "God" and Erica surrendered to her teachings as Erica opened herself to the path of becoming all that she could be. The teachings included listening and following her own true nature. She spent years of inner work processing and removing layer after layer of her conditioning in order to heal her attraction to women. Finally, Erica could no longer contain her feelings and she chose to be with another woman. When she announced her decision, she was rejected by her teacher-mentor. Erica said, "You can imagine how devastated I was to be an outsider. I felt totally untrustworthy, I felt nothing of value or truth and the only way to demonstrate my faithfulness was to return, do what she wanted and to admit I was wrong. I believed I had failed in the only venture that held any value. I was so open on every level to my teacher that when she closed me off, I was shattered, debilitated, and I almost died."

Erica became the scapegoat for the organization's anger and self-righteousness. She suffered from CFIDS, premenopause, and exhaustion. Reflecting back, she said, "I am not surprised at my attraction to a strong woman, as I am still trying to have a relationship with my father." The charismatic, dominant strength of her father was likened to her spiritual teacher's power which mesmerized her; when this was removed, it plunged Erica into the dark abyss of death and rebirth. The dominance of power is not gender specific, as most women have thought for so long.

Erica described her rebirthing event this way, "This happened in order for me to understand that there is a dark side of the universe. My female teacher is the Queen archetype, powerfully controlling; she has yet to face the darkness inside of herself before she knows who she thinks she is." She continued, "I have been on the descent and met the dark feminine and when you get to know her she becomes an ally and you have enormous energy and force available to you. Once you have died to her, you are allowed to create a new life for yourself. My teacher was my universe and I hoped to get the universe through her. When I tried to take my life back, she wouldn't give it back. I needed a new container, one that would not allow others to obliterate mine. Now, I can throw other's feelings into the fire to burn, rather than taking them on. We need to feel the deep part of the dark side of the feminine in order to connect with this energy — to create the pure feminine and to come back out into the world. The dark side actually becomes an ally after we take the risk into the descent. The energy is there after the battle with the self and it is won on behalf of the feminine." As Erica spoke there was a glow of beauty and truth that caught my heart. I felt joined with her feeling, not competitive, or even heartful, but energized with a quality of the wisdom and sacredness of being a women. Her presence was uplifting, and truly healing.

I believe women in every part of the world are emerging from all levels of existence. This is the time for us to be juggled, pushed, and drawn to the depths, to reclaim our feminine energy source, and to bring this energy back to anoint and heal ourselves, each other and Mother Earth.

LEADERSHIP

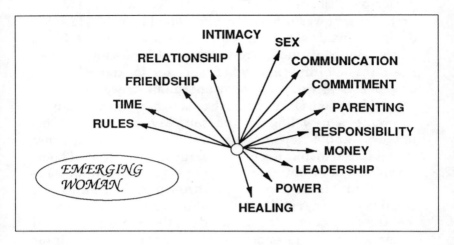

The chart above and the listing on the next page indicate many of the ways the Emerging Woman uses her full powers in leadership.

Emerging Woman — The Authentic Feminine

1. The *Feminine* is set in time; it is a process that goes on in the moment, not forced or planned but within natural rhythms (i.e., in monthly cycles, and in childbirth).
2. The *Feminine* is experienced in friendship; it is the accepting of others no matter who they are.
3. The *Feminine* is at work in relationships; it is a skillful master in making them work.
4. The *Feminine* expresses itself in sex; it is makes it a sacred and a beauteous experience.
5. The *Feminine* reveals intimacy; there is a feeling of closeness without physical touching.
6. The *Feminine* resides in commitment; it reveals the deepest core of her being.
7. The *Feminine* extends in parenting; it guides the child into its own identity.
8. The *Feminine* relates to money; it is the quality and process of creating money.
9. The *Feminine* exerts leadership; it helps others discover and develop their own capabilities.
10. The *Feminine* makes rules; they are made to increase individual freedom rather than impose limits.
11. The *Feminine* is present in communication; it is there to clarify wants, express them clearly, and listen to others for mutual agreement.
12. The *Feminine* acts responsibly; it responds to things when they need to be done without blaming others.
13. The *Feminine* is inherent in process; it follow a series of events rather than concerned in reaching the goal.
14. The *Feminine* instills conservation; it would rather save than destroy or exploit.
15. The *Feminine* is alive in healing; it acknowledges that the decision to get well comes from within the person.

CONCLUSION

Tell me, and I'll forget.
Show me, and I may not remember.
Involve me, and I'll understand.
A Native American saying

As I retrace my steps, and piece together this healing journey, I am amazed at the timing of the events — the healers; the mountain experience; the country move; the revealing dreams; the right books appearing; the discovery of appropriate clinical treatments; experiencing and emerging from the dark night of the soul; the renewed creative energy; the helpful journal writings; and, the women in my research project. The events, unfolding like the making of a patterned quilt, seemed to happen as if planned. The time I spent close to nature forced me to stop, to listen, and join its presence of stillness, wildness, and subtle sounds. With the mountain and earth as my container of energy, I learned that its presence resonated within my body just as Starhawk's litany suggests:

May the animal rise in everyone!
May the voice of the earth roar through us
May we sing for stones and stars
*   and dance as the flames leap and dance*
May we rise!
May every well be a fountain
*   and break free*
*   a shower of sparks*
*   an all-night fiesta*
We have the power to fight for our freedom
*   to erupt volcanic*
*   spouting new lands*
*   forging new tools*
We will not be walking dead
We are earth
*   life is stronger*

we are survivors
animals
we are alive
and life rises! [1]

After my treatments concluded and the women's project was finished, I knew it was time for us to move back to the city. David and I took a car trip along the west coast and we both fell in love with Oregon's beauty and charm. Six weeks later we moved to the northwest and planted our new roots.

David continued traveling and consulting, and I ventured into the community, speaking to groups about my CFIDS experience. I met many people with CFIDS who were seriously ill and who needed support and hope. These people asked for more written material and they encouraged me to write this book.

What is life like now after my illness? Physically I feel good, and I am still learning how to stay healthy. I have not strayed from my CFIDS diet, I limit my activities (I am still learning this one); I do daily exercise on the trampoline, and, I dance, sing and get plenty of rest. If I deviate from this life style my symptoms return. I also have started The Swan Institute, for the Emerging Leader where I counsel, facilitate feminine circles, and do leadership training. By maintaining my healthy life style, I am able to work full time.

My illness has catapulted me to take the next step and do what is important to me. The doors have swung open and I am venturing out. I believe that women often have difficulty responding honestly when asked, "What do you want and what is important to you?" I discovered that women are not often asked this question and they usually respond by feeling guilty, selfish, and self- centered. They also sabotage themselves by saying things like "I can't afford it; my husband wouldn't like it; the economy is bad; I don't want to work that hard; what will people think, and, I am not good enough."

The freedom to personally ask this question, feel safe to reveal the deep hungers, and, then, gather the strength to bolster the dreams into reality is essential to becoming The Emerging Woman. Women have been brainwashed by the authoritarian rule to stay safe, respectable, and cling to their traditional roles and functions. This repression then stifles growth, and it also lowers self esteem.

Are younger women breaking the old traditional ties? Some are, although the establishment's grip is tight on them, too, and they have the same survival fears that run generations deep. I believe that we all (young and old) need to risk asking, "Who and what am I living for? Am I here for the evolution of human kind or just for the old systems? Do I want to die and know I only obliged this authoritarian system, and didn't express my own voice?"

My own first step was to experience my singing dream, so I bought a transportable keyboard and found appropriate music that amplified my story and my women's research. I gave my first presentation to 150 professional women. Although I was terrified, it was a meaningful experience for both me and the audience. The endorphin high was worth every butterfly. I plan to continue to live my dreams!

In writing this book, I reread the fairy tale *Sleeping Beauty* to find out why she fell asleep in the first place. According to the story, there was a glorious celebration before Sleeping Beauty was born. The Wise Women were invited to bestow their magic gifts to the new princess. Since there were only twelve plates, only twelve of the thirteen Wise Women were invited. *"Suddenly the thirteen came in. She wished to avenge herself for not having been invited . . . she cried . . . The King's daughter shall on her fifteenth year will prick herself with a spindle, and fall down dead."*[1] This pronouncement came to pass and everyone in the palace slept for hundreds of years.

Fairy tales can be symbolic maps to give direction to the wisdom and meaning of life. For example, the Wise Women did in fact reign during the matriarchal time and were given high priestess status and carried the inner feminine power for the society. In this tale the spinning/spindle is symbolic of, *"The feminine principle in its skills of weaving destiny and the veil of the world of illusion."*[2] The prick of the finger, and the blood from the wound is the symbol of a sacrifice of the life-rejuvenating force.

My interpretation of the symbols in this fairy tale includes the notion that even before a girl baby is born the feminine has been rejected and cursed. At puberty, the beginning of menstruation and physical changes, young women view themselves differently from young males and realize that the society does not prize them. Thus, throughout her life a woman rejects herself, imitates men and becomes a man's servant. Like Sleeping Beauty, the inner feminine life force energy is sacrificed. Why, then, is the prince able to awaken Sleeping Beauty? I searched for more answers.

In another fairy tale, *Snow-white and the Seven Dwarfs,* Snow-white also goes to sleep. Her stepmother is envious of Snow-white's beauty and attempts to put her to sleep. She is so devious that she dresses as a clothes peddler, and sells Snow White some pretty stay-laces; then, the stepmother laces them so tight that the breath is squeezed out of Snow-white and she falls down as if dead. She is awakened by the seven dwarfs. Then, her stepmother dresses as an old woman and sells Snow-white a beautiful but poisonous comb. Snow-white barely places the comb in her hair and she falls down senseless. *"You paragon of beauty,"* said the wicked woman, *"you are done for now."*[3] But Snow-white is again awakened by the dwarfs. Finally, her stepmother is transformed into a farmer's wife, and sells Snow-white a poisonous apple. To prove the apple is all right, the farmer's wife takes the first bite; when Snow-white bites a piece, however, she falls down dead. This time the dwarfs are unable to awaken her. She does not awaken until the Prince finds her and takes her to his palace. As his servants carry her through the forest they stumble and the sudden jolt dislodges the poisonous apple from Snow-white's throat and she is awakened.

What this fairy tale reveals, is that, as Snow-white falls deeper into the dark hole, her throat, the seat of self expressive power, is closed. The sudden jolt is symbolic of an unexpected life turn, or situation, which awakens her from her victim state. I believe, the way she falls asleep is similar to today's methods. For example, like the pretty stay laces symbol, women's **self esteem** is repressed by not being accepted by the traditional male world; the symbol of the comb signifies that her **self image** is poisoned by the expected traditional women roles; and, the apple symbolizes that her **self knowledge** is undiscovered and unexpressed.

I invite you to take the journey to awaken the feminine and heal the immune system. This system is our defense against illness as it interfaces with both the mind and the body physically, mentally and emotionally. The immune system will break down when we are over-protected; and it will become overloaded when we are too responsible. I believe a woman's immune system is healed when nature's inner feminine presence is felt in the body and her protective power acknowledged. It is interesting that the Latin definition of the word immune means memory. Perhaps, then, the healing of our immune system is to remember what has been repressed. As much as I want to blame everyone and everything for my illness and my unhappiness, I now know that the cultural system rocked me to sleep.

My dream is that there will be many feminine circles all over the world acting as containers to build an energy vortex that will move women into their depths and into their sacred place. As we mirror to each other similar feminine energy patterns, we will be empowered. This self knowledge will breathe into us confidence and self esteem. I believe we can change ourselves and the world around us. We, as women, can help change the world to a more caring place in which to live; to a healthier place in which to raise a family; to an earth that is growing and not decaying, and a people respected and not over-ruled. This power will weave in its way to our daughters and to our daughters' daughters.

Join me as we live this dream together.

APPENDIX A

Phase I Treatment — July 1988 to December 1988

1. Allergy testing & phenal therapy
2. Oxyidative therapy
3. Interferon and staphage lysate (SPL) injections
4. Vitamin, mineral and amino acid therapy
5. Hormonal therapy
6. Weekly Reiki healing sessions outside the clinic -(my idea)
7. Singing - (my idea)

Allergy Testing

The computerized allergy test administered by a technician evaluated all facets of how my body interacted with the environment, and the effect of things I put inside my body. I found this a fascinating and non-invasive testing method. Information about my body's reactions to foods, to supplements and to various allergens was revealed by checking various meridian points on my skin. Although no allergic reaction to environmental pollutants surfaced I was allergic to twenty four foods that worked against me, or that I was allergic to. I learned that most people allergic to foods are generally allergic to a similar set of foods. I was allergic to cane sugar, soy bean, beef, beer, barley malt, cottage cheese, oat, wheat bran, hops, brewers yeast, cow milk, strawberry, whole wheat, honey, cheddar cheese, chocolate, bakers yeast, liver, beet sugar, corn, peanuts, American cheese, mushrooms, tuna fish, and yeast mix. I was advised to stay off of these foods for 9 weeks and was monitored periodically with the phenolic program, a homeopathic remedies program to desensitize and eliminate the allergens to these foods.

Homeopathy is a theory or system of curing diseases

with very minute doses of medicine. It is somewhat difficult and hard to understand because it is the opposite of medicine as we know and understand it. For example, a traditional doctor will usually prescribe drugs that counteract the symptoms the patient is experiencing. If you have a fever, the doctor will give you something to take down the fever. This seems perfectly logical. A homeopathic doctor, however, would approach the problem from the opposite direction. Instead of prescribing a medicine that would reduce the fever, he would give you a tiny dose of a substance, which in large qualities would have caused the type of fever you are experiencing. Although homeopathy has been used for hundreds of years, it has been viewed by modern allelopathic medicine as unscientific and even as quackery. Homeopathy stimulates the natural process of healing in the body, rather than introducing into the body system something that overpowers this natural healing process.

After the third, fourth, and fifth weeks of eliminating the foods I was allergic to, and using the homeopathic desensitization program, I began reintroducing certain foods into my diet. When I completed the desensitization program I was retested on all the foods again. I could now eat the foods on the "bad" list, but after eating one of them, I was cautioned not to eat that same food again for three days. In a month I felt less digestive stress, less flu-like symptoms, and less tiredness, especially in my eyes. I became so aware and sensitive of foods that I could begin to tell whether I was allergic to a food after the first bite. I would immediately get sleepy, my energy level would drop, and my heart would palpitate. What I learned from this experience was to avoid certain foods altogether. I have learned to say no to all sugar based desserts, sandwiches, milk products, and alcohol. And although this has taken much discipline, I am more than willing to avoid these foods because neither do I not want to have the return of these negative symptoms nor another generalized CFIDS relapse.

Part of the problem with food allergies for CFIDS patients is that they have difficulty digesting and assimilating proteins from their foods. With the help of the Heidelberg gastric analysis, an evaluation of the stomach ph and digestive ability, significant information can be obtained for individuals with CFIDS. First, you swallow a pH capsule which is actually a miniature high-frequency transmitter which continuously transmits the pH values from the gastrointestinal tract. The frequencies transmitted are picked up by a belt antenna system worn about the waist.

The receiver then displays the values on a meter and simultaneously records them on a graph. This test is important because many people have very little or no hydrochloric acid in their stomach. The presence of hydrochloric acid and pepsin in the stomach is essential to initiate digestion of food. The normal stomach contains hydrochloric acid, pepsin, mucin and intrinsic factors which are necessary to absorb vitamin B-12. The acid and pepsin initiate digestion and work to change proteins into amino acids. The proteins are converted by enzymatic action into amino acids and sent to the small intestine to be absorbed into the blood stream.

The results of this test proved that my digestive problems were connected to having very little secretion of this digestive acid. This meant that I was absorbing very little protein into the blood stream of my body. Why is the lack of protein absorption so important? Because proteins are the main structural component of tissues and organs. Protein manufacture is essential to all aspects of growth and repair of cells.

Oxidative Therapy

My food allergies were tested at the same time I began to have hydrogen peroxide dripped into my veins. Hydrogen peroxide contains an enzyme (catalase) which, when exposed to the blood, or other body fluids, chemically spits into oxygen and water. The body uses oxidation as its first line of defense against bacteria, viruses, yeast, parasites. Even breathing oxygen is an oxidative process.

Oxidation is also a part of a system which helps the body regulate all living cell membranes. It is a hormonal regulator, necessary for our bodies to produce several hormonal substances such as estrogen, progesterone, and thyroid. It is important in the regulation of blood sugar and the production of energy in all cells. It helps regulate certain chemicals necessary to operate the brain and nervous system. And, fundamentally important for people with CFIDS, oxygen is used in regulating the immune system.

Injections of hydrogen peroxide were first reported being used by doctors in the 1920s. Oxygen therapy is a new use of an old treatment for treating such diseases as allergies, arthritis, asthma, cancer, candida, colds, diabetes, flu, heart problems, hepatitis, herpes, lukemia, MS, and ulcers. Sedentary lifestyles, poor foods, lack of exercise, and shallow breathing of polluted air are contributing factors that have created a chronic low oxygen condition in our cells. The viruses and microbes (in flu, colds, AIDS, arterial plaque and cancer cells) live best in low oxygen environments. If the cells are flooded with oxygen, however, these viruses and microbes can't live. This condition of oxygen flooding creates an anaerobic condition. This means if the oxygen level is raised and the cell environments are supplied with oxygen, then the viruses and microbes will die and the body waste products will be burned up.

For my oxygen treatment I was given a weak, but pure hydrogen peroxide placed in a sugar water solution. After the hydrogen peroxide solution was dripped into my veins, I then had an amino acid I.V. dripped into my veins with nutritional supplements of a B-complex, Vitamin C, B-12, B-5, B-6, potassium chloride, germanium, DMSO and calcium. The solution was administered into a large vein, usually in my arm, over a period of 3 hours. How long the drip took depended on both the amount of solution and my overall condition on that particular day. The drip treatments are generally given about once a week, but in my case, with an extreme chronic illness, I sometimes had them three times a week. Generally 10 to 15 treatments are needed, depending on the condition of the patient and type of illness being treated. I was treated with 40 hydrogen peroxide drips over a five month period.

With the food allergy program, revised diet, and receiving drips three times a week, I began the healing process in earnest. This was a much different experience than just lying in bed feeling depressed and sorry for myself. I was either at the clinic or in bed recovering from the prescribed series of treatments. David would drive me to the clinic and I would slowly hobble in to a large room filled with twenty large recliners. Resting on a recliner I was then hooked to the oxygen drip. Because I had so many drips the nurse occasionally had trouble finding new veins in my arms for the needle. If she used the old place too often, my vein might collapse. Sometimes I felt pain when the solution entered my arm because the B vitamins would burn the tissue and veins. At the end of a week my arm and hands often would be a mass of black and blue marks from the needle incisions breaking blood vessels. My body would give off a smell for hours afterwards from the DMSO that was added to the oxygen drip. On the trip home I would often feel worse than when I went to the clinic.

Yes, beginning the healing process for CFIDS isn't necessarily easy, especially for someone who has been sick a long while. Essentially, because my body was breaking down and dying, I was working hard to get it back on a healthy course. To get one's body back on track takes enormous personal effort and commitment. I told myself that there was a battle going on between the viruses and the oxygen. I wanted the oxygen to win — viruses do not not like to live in an oxygen-rich environment. With the stiffness in my joints, the flu-like symptoms, the chronic low energy, and depression, on top of all the other symptoms I truly doubted that I was getting better. Plus, I was feeling somewhat guilty about all, the time, energy, and money we had expended on me. I was heartened, finally, when a wise and loving friend suggested, that I was in a "healing crisis." She said, "What you're experiencing is normal in the healing process — the darkness before the dawn." I wasn't getting worst, rather I was at the critical point — at the crisis — of breaking through to the light of real healing. Again, in the midst of the struggle and darkness I received a measure of hope. "Maybe," I thought, "I am going to get better after all."

"But why does this healing have to be so difficult?" I kept asking myself. I had decided to live, I had something to look forward to, but why was the healing so slow? I had thought the healing would happen instantly, but it didn't.

When I first went to the clinic, I believed that in four months I would be on my way to living an active, normal, and productive life. Well, it didn't happen for me that way. And, it doesn't seem to happen for most Chronic Fatigue victims. I remember one instance trying to visit with a friend of David's. All I could do was curl up on the couch and lie there. I didn't have enough energy to even look at her or converse in an orderly manner. Another time I woke up after having a drip the day before, and I couldn't get out of bed. David was already in town so I telephoned him to find out what to do. We decided that I should crawl down the stairs and take a warm bath. After the warm energizing bath, I could get up, walk, and finally get something nourishing to eat. I assume many of these strange physical reactions happened because the virus was being eliminated by the added oxygen, and my immune system was being fed supplements in order to fight off the virus. This healing crisis was like a constant battle going on inside my entire body. These were tough days for me.

Yet instinctively I knew the new diet and the oxygen treatments were the right processes for my healing. I believe what is needed from each of us who has suffered from Chronic Fatigue Immune Dysfunction Syndrome is to learn to trust ourselves first and then if necessary get advice from medical resources. I made the decisions about what felt best rather than relying totally on what others said was the right plan for my healing. Even with my "alternative" doctor I had to fight and say "no" to suggestions that didn't feel right for me. *Over and over I learned that the only way I could get better was to take charge of my own healing.* I came to sessions with the doctor with lists of questions. I debated with him on diagnosis, proper treatments, and interpretation of my medical tests. By choosing to live and survive this insidious disease, I found that taking an active role in my recovery was critical. I became proactive on my own behalf.

As I look back on my treatment, I believe that the oxidation drips were one of the significant treatments in the physical part of my recovery. Fortunately, my insurance covered these expensive treatments. For more information and to find where you can locate a physician trained in oxidative therapy, write to International Bio-

Oxidative Medicine Foundation P.O. Box 61767, Dallas/ Fort Worth, Texas, 75261, USA.

Injections

In the immune system are lymphokines such as interferon or interleukin. These lymphokines are used to fight infection and regulate the immune system. Lymphokines are capable of stimulating the reproductive capability of cells of the immune system, while at the same time impairing the reproductive capability of the invading viruses. As part of my treatment program I had injections of interferon once a week to strengthen my immune system.

Another injection that the doctor prescribed was staphage lysate (SPL). I had these injections once a week for 2 months. SPL is is also an augmenting agent in cancer therapy. This drug also activates natural killer cells in the body as well as other natural effector cells. SPL enables the immune system to respond more effectively to viruses.

Vitamin, Mineral and Amino Acid Therapy

With all the many bottles of tablets and capsules on the counter, our kitchen looked like a health food store. Before visting the Preventative Medical Clinic I knew that my body needed extra vitamin and mineral supplements, but I was never quite sure which ones. At the clinic I was given a helpful education on the value of vitamins and minerals. Rather than just popping pills, I observed my reactions to various supplements, as well as noticing how well different dosages and combinations of supplements worked, or didn't work. The supplements that had the greatest positive effect on reducing my CFIDS symptoms were the following:

1. Antioxidants/Immune Enhancers
CoQ10
Aerobic 07 (liquid oxygen)

> Germanium
> LEM-Shitaki mushrooms

The Shitake mushroom is a particularly potent natural supplement that acts as an immune system stimulator and possesses anti-viral properties. LEM is an extract from immature shitaki mushrooms and lentian (an extract from the mushroom's fruit body). Both LEM and lentian appear to stimulate immune responses but differ in their anti-viral properties. LEM is effective in restoring and bolstering immune response by stimulating lymphocytes and macrophages responsible for the immune system's defense against bacteria, viruses, tumor cells and toxins. It has been effective in stimulating production of antibodies to hepatitis B and to improving liver function. The positive thing about LEM is that it may interfere with reverse transcriptaise activity which is in the retrovirus of AIDS, and other retroviruses.

2. Minerals

> Calcium/magnesium
> Multi-mineral tablets

3. Vitamins

> Folic acid
> Vitamin C
> B-6
> Beta carotene
> Multi-vitamin tablets
> AKG

4. Glandular

> Iron
> Hemocrine complex
> Thyroid
> Estrogen replacement therapy

5. Digestive Aids
   Betaine hydochloride
   Lipamase
   Pancreas
   Acidophilus

6. Amino Acids
   Glycine
   Cysteine
   Lysine
   Phenylalanine

A bio-chemist at the clinic evaluated my digestive problems. Many CFIDS patients have digestive problems. The amino proteins bio-chemistry panel was helpful because it evaluated and pointed out the degree to which the aminproteins were functioning in my body and indicated which amino proteins needed to be supplemented.

Hormonal Therapy
   Soon after beginning both the oxygen drips and taking the glandular thyroid my throat started to loosen up. For months my throat felt squeezed by a steel vise. Further tests revealed that I also had Hashimoto's thyroiditis, an autoimmune disease, in addition to the CFIDS. Any kind of autoimmune reactions may be set off by infection, tissue injury, or emotional trauma. This autoimmune disease is often a secondary problem of the general immune system breaking down, and the presence of a virus in the nervous system. I believe that, in my case, the months of extreme emotional reaction, fear, and trauma contributed to the onset of this disease. Because the chemical thyroid that is usually prescribed by traditional physicians creates a dependency on the chemical thyroid, I was given the glandular thyroid to support the current lack of thyroid. This helped build up the gland's capacity to produce its own secretions once again.

Reiki Treatments

Healing is a natural process. Our bodies have built-in means to restore health and balance to various internal systems when they are threatened. Through understanding the way the body and mind work in harmony to facilitate healing in oneself or another person, medicine people, healers, and doctors throughout the centuries discovered that they are as much a part of the healing process as are the plants or drugs they use. The energy of the healer is an important ingredient in the patient's return to health. It is believed that the giving of positive "energy," good feelings, or hopefulness from the healer to the patient can increase the patient's vitality and speed up one's recovery no matter what physical manipulation or medicine is given. Natural healers are those who either have a strong natural link with their own inner source of energy, or who have worked and practiced to develop such a link.

Healers can be trained as doctors, or they can be lay persons who have discovered this healing gift. Once this link is established and functioning properly, the healer has a supply of vital, universal energy that can be shared with others in need. This vitality can be directed to patients in a variety of ways to help them overcome whatever internal or external factors have put them out of touch with their own source of strength. This "energy boost" from a healer then frees the natural healing powers of the patient's mind and body to correct the imbalances.

It seems that everyone is born with a personal healing energy envelope around them. We use this energy to heal broken bones and fight infections. The Chinese developed the system of acupuncture based on this energy field in the body, calling the energy "chi." Many indigenous peoples from around the world describe this energy in many ways.

Shamans and medicine people learned to call on the spirit forces of nature to help them use this energy for healing. The Greeks used both sound and color therapy to help activate these healing energy fields. Dance and martial arts practices were developed in order to learn how to control this energy in the body.

Outside our personal energy field is a vast and limitless sea of universal healing energy. This is a balanced, resonating, harmonizing energy available to everyone. This vast field of energy is integrated and it has no positive or negative charge to it. It is complete and ready to be utilized. Reiki (pronounced ray-key) is one such healing method for people who have learned to access this abundance of natural universal energy. Reiki is a Japanese word meaning "universal life energy." In simplest terms Reiki is a method of "laying hands" on a person who is ill; the universal energy is transfered through their hands to the body of the sick person. A complete Reiki treatment can last one to two hours. The receiver of the treatment either sits or lies down, clothed, and the Reiki practitioner places his or her hands on the body corresponding to the major organs, and various glands. There is often an experience of warmth from the practitioner's hands.

Reiki was established as a practice in the 1800s in Japan, by Dr. Mikao Usui. Dr. Usui was president of a Christian school in Kyoto, Japan. When he was asked by his students to explain and demonstrate the healing power of Jesus, he didn't know how to respond. Dr. Usui resigned from his position and began an intensive search to discover the secrets of the healing miracles ascribed to Christ and Buddha. After seven years he found what he was seeking in a 2500 year old Sanskrit sutra. The sutras are principles and teachings in Hindu and Buddhist literature. Dr. Usui began to practice the healing hands-on technique, he found in the sutra, with amazing results. A lineage of three other Reiki masters have passed on the way to use this healing energy from the universe to thousands of Reiki practitioners around the world.

Reiki became a significant part of my healing treatment along with the traditional allopathic and homeopathic methods. At least once a week I received a hands-on treatment by a local Reiki practitioner, and I found that more than my physical body was being healed by this universal energy.

Singing

Three months into this treatment plan, I was captivated by a woman's picture in a course catalog. Without a second thought, I signed up for a course in chanting by Jill Purce. I love to sing, and intuitively I know that this kind of singing would be good for me. Although I had previous experience with Buddhist chanting, I didn't learn until I arrived at the retreat that the instructor's method would be a form of Tibetan overtone chanting. Because I had never heard of this type of chanting, I should have been more cautious about attending, but I was so taken by the warm feeling of this woman when I met her that I decided to endure the nearly three days in the rustic mountain retreat center. To my surprise, however, I not only lasted for the weekend but I decided to remain for the week to experience the in-depth chanting course. I stayed ten days away from my food, my treatments, and my familiar routine. I was flabbergasted! At first, I rested in the afternoons, and had some difficulty sleeping on the futon beds at night because my muscles and joints were so sore. But as the week progressed my body was less sore, I slept better, and I could make it through some days without napping in the afternoon. I felt more pleasantly energized from the chanting than anything else I had done for my treatment.

Jill Purce is an incredible teacher of sound. Like the Reiki treatment that uses the hands of one to transfer universal healing energy to another, Jill taught me the magical healing qualities of the universal energy that comes through sound. On the first day she told us why she was teaching the course. She said, "The healing and transformative power of sound is what interests me the most." She talked about the creative power of sound, and how it is one of the most effective ways of getting beyond separation of ourselves from God, or from another person. "The separation of *us* and *not us* is the separation which all traditions try to overcome so that we can be in a state of unity," she explained.

What was this process of using sound that made me feel so much better? First, in the overtone chanting you make a sound as separate notes over and above the main note which you are singing. This is a magical thing to accomplish because you begin to have a sense that you are evoking a higher vibration of energy. The technique of overtone chanting comes from Buddhist monks in Tibet. Tibet is a very old medieval, spiritual culture that has survived the modern age. The Tibetans talk about the human being in three ways, of body, of voice, and of mind. The position for 'body' is in the head, the 'voice' is in the throat, and, the position of 'mind' is in the heart. For Tibetans there is no distinction between mind and brain, as there is in the West. They believe the voice acts as an intermediary between the subtle realm of mind and the heart.

The voice, then, is seen as a bridge between the material and the non-material world. According to our instructor, Jill Purce, "If you can liberate the voice, then you can liberate a human being." The voice is our means of expression. It is the way in which our breath is made conscious.

Our breath is the way we have of exchanging ourselves with the world. We breathe the world in and we breathe ourselves out into the world. The breath is in a constant relationship which continues on a mostly unconscious level. With the use of the voice, however, the breath becomes conscious. Jill first taught us how to breath consciously. The second thing she taught us was to not just make a sound, but to listen after the sound so as to complete a circuit of attention between sound and no sound. In this circuit of attention, we are able to go beyond the thinking mind. Lastly, Jill had us experience listening and making sounds at the same time.

We were taught how to use sound to liberate ourselves from the pattern of anxieties in our lives. She emphasized that the persistence of negative thought patterns causes stress which affects our emotions and general body energy. Accumulated stress then brings about material changes at our body's weakest points. The longer the stress remains lodged at these weak points in the body, the faster the body breaks down and we get sick. With metaphors that show the relationship of sound to health, we hear and use phrases like "being sound in body and mind," or having something "ring true," or being "in tune with our bodies." An important part of our learning during the week-long retreat was to find our own unique body sound. Jill explained that finding sound and using it could help us maintain our own health and sanity. Because each person, she said, has their own distinct sound, we spent time exploring the depth, power, and healing of sound within us.

The indigenous medicine people of North America would ask four questions to any of their people who were ill: "When was the last time that you sang?"; "When was the last time you danced?"; "When was that last time you enjoyed the enchantment of story telling?"; and, "When was the last time you experienced silence?" Singing, dancing, story telling, and silence are called the four healing salves. I recommend that you make sounds, a healing salve as a part of your treatment plan. As you sing, fill your stomach with air in addition to just your lungs, in order to have a deeper foundation to give to your sound. Then release the breath with a musical sound using the A-E-I-O-U vowels — they are considered sacred sounds by many traditions. I felt better and better as I got more grounded in my bodily earth energy of sound. It seemed as though I was touching my soul when I sang or chanted. I returned home from the mountain retreat with renewed hope, with the healing energy of sound, and with the knowledge of how to incorporate chanting into my treatment plan.

APPENDIX B

Phase II Treatment Plan — November to May 1989

1. Acupuncture and auto son treatments.
2. Self administered B-12 shots.
3. Vitamin, mineral and amino acid therapy.
4. Monthly meetings with the doctor.
5. Weekly Reiki healing sessions, outside the clinic .
6. Progoff journal writing and dream work.

1. Acupuncture and Auto Son Treatments

Acupuncture and acupressure were two of the first therapies from oriental medicine to establish themselves in the Western hemisphere. As far back as ancient Neolithic times the Chinese used needles of bone or bamboo, inserting them into the body's many energy points or meridians. Today, the acupuncturist uses needles of processed stainless steel.

Acupressure uses the same principles as acupuncture, but rather than using needles to activate the energy points, pressure from the fingers is applied to these points.

Acupuncture and acupressure hold the theory that there are two flows of energy, called yin and yang, which exist in the body. This flow of energy is known as the Life Force or Chi. This Chi energy is understood to be part of everything we do, think or feel. When yin and yang energies flow freely, and are in balance with each other, they produce what we know as health. When the flow is blocked or unbalanced, disease results. The Chinese discovered that this vital energy circulates through the body in the same way as the blood flows. The channels of this energy are called meridians.

For people with Epstein-Barr virus, and, later, Chronic Fatigue Immune Dysfunction Syndrome, acupuncture had been the most widely recommended alternative treatment. When in the early stages of my illness, I had an acupuncture treatment and found that it seemed to make my symptoms worse, I discontinued this method. Only later did I learn that this negative reaction is one of the first signs of toxicity in the body; these toxins need to be worked through and released for the healing to go forward.

As I was coming to the end of my I.V. drips, the clinic staff had started to use auto son injections to see if they would help CFIDS patients. I too, was eager to see how they would work for me. First, the nurse would take some blood from my finger, then the homeopathic doctor would mix selected homeopathic remedies into my blood sample. The nurse would then inject the mixture back into my stomach meridian (which is the acupuncture point in the side of the knees). The homeopathic remedies were for my thyroid, Epstein Barr-virus, anemia, arthritis, and allergies. After the treatments I would feel a little more energized. I do believe that the auto son injections helped boost my immune resistance to the particular problems I was having.

While I was undergoing a series of these treatments, *Chronic Fatigue Syndrome, The Hidden Epidemic,* by Jesse A. Stoff, M.D., and Charles R. Pellegrino, Ph.D, was published. The authors list and describe how to use homeopathic remedies for the Epstein-Barr virus, the thyroid, and the adrenals. When I showed the list of remedies to the clinic staff, they decided to try them on me for a generalized treatment for CFIDS.

After the acupuncturist had first completed the session and found my weakest meridian point, the auto son solution was then injected into that point. At first, I felt an increased jolt to my energy system for a day or two after the treatment. In the twice-monthly treatments that followed for the next several months, I noticed a gentle, subtle longer-lasting improvement.

Singing

I also joined a choir which sang sacred, classical, and some modern music. This was indeed music for my soul. At first I wondered if I would make it through the two hours of rehearsal, but once again the sound and the active participation kept my energy going. This regular weekly singing maintained a "sound" discipline within a group context. I continued to practice on my own, chanting at home in the way I learned from Jill Purce.

Intensive Journal Writing and Dream Writing

In 1966 Ira Progoff created the Intensive Journal model. Progoff's book, *At a Journal Workshop,* has served as an instrument for learning his method and for keeping an in-depth personal journal. The importance of Progoff's method is that it actively extends one's life experience. It works on many levels that enable a person to crystallize not only the present situation, but the past as well and thus be in a better position to make decisions and move into the future. According to Progoff, Intensive Journal carries the dynamic of the inner process by going into the underlying stream embodying one's own inner source in a way to get a mirroring and a feedback effect. The journal is divided into a number of sections; these compartments are like a filing system for the psyche. I found that the sustained use of the journal for several months gave me feedback from these various sections. This helped me have an overall perspective of my illness, especially when I thought there was no movement forward in my healing process. My daily journal provided accessible feedback on my process that may have been too intangible or elusive from just a dream analysis.

Dreams, however, speak to us in a right-brained manner about our life. They give us messages about our life purpose in patterns we are unaware of, and they also reflect tensions, anxieties, and desires that we are not yet conscious of. The Intensive Journal has two separate sections for dream work, the dream log and dream enlargements. The dream log is a daily logging of the contents of dreams. I also compared my daily log with my dream log to notice synchronistic connection of my inner and outer life experiences. I applied what Progoff calls the Twilight Dreaming — noticing a series of dreams until I felt part of their rhythm; then other scenes and images often reappeared to help me learn more from the dream-life process. According to Progoff, The Twilight Dreaming section of the journal can offer tangible information about one's life. I found the whole process of the *Intensive Journal* writing an essential part of my healing from CFIDS.

APPENDIX C

Phase III Treatment Plan —August 1989 to May 1990

1. Hydrocortisone, and DHEAS
2. Massage
3. Colonics
4. Herbalism
5. Candida diet (2 months)
6. Music-piano and singing
7. Creating a research project
8. Exercise
9. Journal writing

Hydrocortisone and DHEAS

I took 10 ml of hydrocortisone once a day. I also took 150 ml of DHEAS each day. DHEAS (dehydroeplandrosterone sulfate) is another hormone produced by the adrenal gland. Researchers at the University of California at San Diego found that older men who had high levels of the hormone were less likely to die of heart disease than were men with low levels of the hormone. Researchers are finding that a higher levels of DHEAS in the system is a way of helping people to live longer.

I responded very quickly to this treatment and within two months I felt like my old self. In fact, I went off this medication nine months later. A very simple way you can tell if you have adrenal problems is to bend over and touch your toe. When you rise back up if you feel dizzy there may be a problem with your adrenals. Also, another way to identify adrenal insufficiency is to take your blood pressure twice. Take it once when you are lying down and then again right after you sit up. If there is a large discrepancy in the measurement of your blood pressure it may indicate adrenal malfunctioning.

Colonic Irrigation

A month after taking hydrocortisone and DHEAS, I heard that still small voice within again telling me I needed to have some colonics. I felt clogged up and full in my intestines; I needed to get cleaned out. I had experienced a few colonics in my life that had really helped reduce pressure in the colon and return me to more regular bowel movements. I can't say enough about the value I received from colonics in this phase of my healing. Because my body had been very inactive, there was an accumulation of fecal matter that was crusted in my colon. During the last nine months of my healing, which I call the purification process, I had fifty colonics.

What is a colonic? First, the word "constipate" means to press together. So constipation is a condition in which one's feces are packed together. There are two types of constipation. One type is present when the feces that pass from the body are overly packed together. Another type of constipation is present when old hardened feces actually stick to the walls of the colon and do not pass out with the regular bowel movements. Few people have any idea how many old, hardened feces are chronically present in the colon.

The residues of digested food empty from the small intestines into the colon in liquid form. Muscular contractions of the colon move this material towards the rectum. The longer the material remains in the colon, the more moisture is absorbed from it, and the more dry and pressed together the feces become. The old feces may build up in pockets and/or may coat the entire length of the colon, as well as the small intestines. They do not evacuate from the body with ordinary bowel movements but require special methods in order to dissolve them in the colon and pass them out via the rectum.

Colonic irrigation is based on the same principle as that of an enema. Although it requires more complicated equipment and affects a larger area of the body than an enema, the procedure is simple. For a varying period of time water is injected into the rectum at body temperature. The water then flows out of the rectum carrying fecal matter through a second tube. Irrigation is more effective than an enema because it reaches above the normal defecation area, into the descending and transverse colon. As the water is washed in and out of the colon it detaches any old fecal matter that adheres to the walls. During irrigation many of the normal digestive bacteria are washed out of the colon.

The practitioner instructed me to implant acidophilus into my rectum before and after each colonic. Any time you take antibiotics, or are under chronic stress, or take birth control pills, hydrocortisone, or take estrogen replacement pills, the good bacteria in the colon is reduced. Replenishing the system every day by taking acidophilus is a must for anyone with an immune problem as well as those using antibiotics or taking birth control pills. The destruction of good bacteria in our colons is a major contributor to poor absorption of nutrients. The implanting process I used after the colonics was an enema with a solution of the acidophilus bacteria in it.

Because CFIDS reduces energy and vitality, a person may not have the stamina to go through the colonic process. From my experience, I believe the time to use colonics is in the final phases of the healing process, when one's energy is returning to normal levels. I think I would not have had enough energy to manage them early in my illness. For me it was a final purification process that removed the last of all the toxins from my body after years of being so sedentary.

The reason I continued to take so many colonics is that I could feel the reduction of specific chronic symptoms. First, I experienced a noticeable increase in energy the day after a session, and, the arthritic swelling and pain in my joints reduced markedly. I had also learned from my research that Addison's disease creates chronic constipation. I am convinced that colon irrigation is an important part of the treatment process for those with CFIDS; this procedure removes toxins and purifies the body so that the natural systems of immunity and defense can restore natural balance to the system.

During the colonic sessions, I noticed all kinds of gas, and very old fecal matter being removed via the glass exit tube. Because gas was being created in my colon, especially after eating lamb and beef, I soon eliminated red meat from my diet. I learned that the presence of gas inhabits the colon from eliminating body wastes and contributes to the buildup of fecal matter.

After the first few colonic sessions I went home nauseated, exhausted, and achy. The next day I would wake up exhausted and with a headache. This was particularly uncomfortable when I was having three to four sessions a week. However, when I had just one or two sessions a week, I found that a day or two afterward my energy would increase measurably. This encouraged me to continue with the colonics even though the process was less than pleasant.

Massage and Bodybrushing

Once a week I would scheduled a massage from a massage therapist right before the colonic session. The massage would relax me for the colonic and increase the flow of blood into those parts of my body that had been chronically sore. The positive mental and emotional nurturing from the massage therapist gave my body a feeling of pleasure and comfort. Also, being in a safe and supportive environment helped to rebuild and restore my self esteem. When chronically sick for a long period of time, you often lose respect and liking for your own body. To restore a positive image about my body was an important part of my purification process.

One simple technique I learned, to help stimulate the lymph system, was to do body brushing. Before stepping into the shower or bath, use a dry bath brush to lightly brush the entire body. The direction of the brushing should always be downwards toward the lower abdomen in one continuous stroke then brush down the neck toward the mid part of the body. Finally brush up the arms, legs and buttocks toward the lower abdomen. Brush across the top of the shoulders and upper back toward the abdomen. This skin brushing should be performed once or twice a day. I was advised to use a long-handled, bath-type brush. It is essential that it contain natural vegetable bristles. This brushing process helps remove lymph mucoid that is stimulated and brought to the surface of the skin.

Juicing Fresh Foods

I was encouraged by my doctor to get a juicer. Because of my digestive problems, he suggested letting my digestive system rest. Raw juiced vegetables require little digestion in the stomach compared with cooked food and fruit juices which remain in the stomach for a shorter period of time than whole fruits. Raw vegetables, he said, go through the digestive system largely as bulk, and are not fermentative, as are cooked foods. Vegetable juices and fresh fruit juices require no work on the part of the digestive system; they are absorbed directly into the blood and can be utilized by the weakest of stomachs. I was cautioned not to liquify the food but to juice them because the liquefiers produces cellulose and pulp which are hard to digest. With a juicer the solids are eliminated and you have only the pure concentrated juice. He said, "You wouldn't think of eating a table full of raw vegetables, but your system may be starving for the minerals, vitamins, and enzymes contained in that table full of raw vegetables. The minerals, vitamins, and enzymes can be used by our bodies only when they are consumed as part of the whole food in which they occur, and the best way to get them into our bodies is through fresh juice."

In doing some reading on juicing vegetables I found that certain combination of juices had specific application to different parts of the body and to different diseases and problems. For example, the best juices for my anemia and arthritis were a mixture of carrot, celery, beet, and cucumber. To stimulate and help the colon function better I added an apple to any of the juice combinations. To reduce constipation I drank a combination of carrot, apple, celery, spinach and grape juice. To flush the liver I juiced a combination of carrots, beets, parsley, cucumbers, dandelions and radishes. One of the best all around purification juices was watermelon. The red fruit part with the seeds, not the rind, helped to clean out the intestinal track. I used this juice daily when I was going through the series of colonics. When those with CFIDS or any other auto immune disease are fighting hard to rebuild their immune systems, it is useful to give the digestive system a rest. It is also valuable to give the metabolic system a direct injection of vitamins and minerals that doesn't require the energy that is taken through digestion.

Herbalism

Using specific plants to treat various problems and ailments in the body goes back beyond recorded history. Indigenous peoples from around the world are caretakers of this earth-centered herbal wisdom. Many of our modern drugs are a direct result of chemically analyzing some of these native plants. Quinine, the oldest drug treatment for malaria, was discovered by observing natives in the jungle chewing a particular plant. The researchers wondered why the natives didn't get malaria while the white people did. A so-called "witch doctor" told the researchers that his people specifically chewed the plant to protect them from getting the "fever."

Through trial and error, individuals learned that certain plants applied externally or taken internally had specific healing properties. There are records of herbal medicine being used back to 1500 B.C. in the western world. Ancient records of Chinese herbal medicine indicate a sophisticated understanding of the chemical properties in plants, their effect on different parts of the body, and their use in a wide variety of physical maladies. Herbalism is the oldest and certainly one of the best established of the "alternative therapies."

Herbal medicine is best described as the art and science of restoring health by using remedies originating from plants. These remedies are in many cases just as powerful as orthodox drugs.

Candida Diet

In May of 1989 the Preventive Medical Clinic in Sacramento, California closed its doors. I was stunned, as were many of the other patients who had come from all over the country to get alternative medical help. I went back to the preventive medical doctor I had seen in the early stages of my illness. I informed him of my progress and told him of the white candida emerging from my body during the colonic sessions. He put me on a candida diet and instructed me to take a particular over-the-counter pill, paramicrociden, a citrus seed extract. I followed this specific candida diet plan for two months. Some of the key items on this diet were lemons, limes, unsweetened cranberry juice, fresh cheese, yeast-free grains; then, proteins such as meat, eggs, tofu and legumes; and all vegetables and nuts except peanuts. This is just a partial food list; it is best to contact your health care physician who that will personalize a diet for you.

Candida may cause a thick, white discharge from the vagina, and/or itching in the vaginal area, which may then cause a burning sensation when passing urine. However, when the body's resistance is lowered with any immune disease like AIDS or CFIDS the yeast fungus may multiply and overgrow the intestinal track as well as the vagina.

Many traditional doctors are skeptical of candida in the intestinal track, but alternative doctors argue that its fatiguing effect on the body is a symptom of lowering the defense of the immune system. Clearing up candida in the system is an important purification and rebuilding of the body to reestablish health and build resistance to viruses and micro organisms. Whether one has CFIDS or some other immune disease, following a prescribed method to clear candida from the system will help increase your energy, as well as build your resistance to colds, flus and other bugs that abound in our daily world.

Exercise

As I started feeling better, I began to jump on a trampoline jumper at least five minutes a day. Now I am up to a half an hour a day. I was told that jumping was one of the best ways to keep the lymph system circulating. The lymph system is formed in tissue spaces all over the body and is gathered into small vessels which carry toxins out of the body. The lymph nodes produce lymphocytes and monocytes, and these act as filters to keep particle matter, especially bacteria, from gaining entrance to the blood stream. Since CFIDS creates dysfunction to the immune system I wanted to stimulate their production in many different ways. The jumping activity was both an invigorating and practical way to accomplish this purpose. I would put on some of my favorite music and combine my singing and sound therapy with the physical exercise. Daily singing and jumping picked me up both physically and emotionally.

CREATING THE RESEARCH PROJECT

The details of this project are discussed in Part IV.

Notes
The footnoted references for each chapter are listed first and then followed by primary sources.

INTRODUCTION

1. Barks, Coleman & Bly, Robert. *Night and Sleep.* Cambridge: Yellow Moon Press, 1981. "Across The Doorsill."

- Sams, Jamie and Carson, David. *Medicine Cards The Discovery of Power Through The Ways of Animals.* New Mexico: Bear and Company, 1988.

PART I

1. Calhoun, Marcy. *Are You Really Too Sensitive? How to Develop & Understand Your Sensitivity as the Strength it is.* Nevada City, CA: Blue Dolphin Press, 1987 pp. 31-32.

- Leviton, Richard. "What Does Illness Mean?" *Yoga Journal* (November/December 1991).

PART II

- AMA. *The American Medical Association Encyclopedia of Medicine.* New York: Random House, 1989.

- Boly, Williams. "Raggedy Ann Town." *Hippocrates* (July/August 1987).

- Conant, Susan. *Living With Chronic Fatigue. New Strategies for Coping with and Conquering CFS.* Texas: Taylor Publishing Co. 1990.

- DeFreitas, Hilliard, Brendan. "Association Of An HTSV-II-Like Virus with CFIDS. *The CFIDS Chronicle* (Spring, 1991).

- Feiden, Karyn. *Hope and Help for Chronic Fatigue Syndrome*. New York: Prentice Hall Press, 1990.

- King, Sheila. *Reiki House* (August 1991).

- Ostrom, Neenyah. "What Really Killed Gilda Radner?" New York: *The New Magazine*, Inc., 1991.

- Stoff, Jesse A;, Pellegrino, Charles; *Chronic Fatigue Syndrome, The Hidden Epidemic*. New York: Random House, 1988.

PART III

1. Ostrom, Neenyah. "What Really Killed Gilda Radner?" New York: *The New Magazine*, Inc., 1991. p. 121.

2. Williams, Linda. "Stalking a Shadowy Assailant." *Time* (May 14, 1990). p.66

3. Landay, Alan; Jessop, Carol; Lennette, Evelyne; Levy, Jay. "Chronic fatigue syndrome: clinical condition associated with immune activation." *Lancet*. (Vol. 338. No. 8769. Saturday 21 Sept. 1991). p. 711.

- Cowley, Geoffrey. "Chronic Fatigue Syndrome, A Modern Medical Mystery." *Newsweek* (November 12, 1990). pp. 62-70.

- CFIDS Teleconference, Portland, Oregon. November, 1991.

- DeFreitas, Elaine; Hilliard, Brendan; Cheney, Paul; Bell, David. "Retroviral sequences related to human T-lymphotropic virus type II in patients with chronic fatigue immune dysfunction syndrome." Proc. Natl. Acad. Sci. USA. (Vol. 88. April 1991). pp. 2922-2926.

- Fisher, Gregg, Straus, Stephen, Cheney, Paul, Oleske, James. *Chronic Fatigue Syndrome, A Victim's Guide To Understanding, Treating, & Coping With This Debilitating Illness.* New York: Time Warner Books, 1987.

- Hendler, Sheldon. *The Oxygen Breakthrough 30 Days to an Illness-Free Life.* New York: William Morrow & Co., 1989.

- Klimas, Nancy; Salvato, Fernando; Morgan, Robert; Fletcher, Mary Ann. "Immunologic Abnormalities in Chronic Fatigue Syndrome." *Journal of Clinical Microbiology,* (June 1990). p. 1403-1410.

- Landay, Alan; Jessop, Carol; Lennette, Evelyne; Levy, Jay. "Chronic fatigue syndrome: clinical condition associated with immune activation." *Lancet.* (Vol. 338. No. 8769. Saturday 21 Sept. 1991).

- Poesnecker, G.E. *Adrenal Syndrome, The Disease No Doctor Wants To Treat.* PA: Humanitarian Publishing Company, 1988.

- Solomon, Neil. *Sick & Tired of being Sick & Tired.* New York: Wynwood Press, 1989.

- Stoff, Jesse A.; Pellegrino, Charles. *Chronic Fatigue Syndrome, The Hidden Epidemic.* New York: Random House, 1988.

- Wilkinson, Steve. *Chronic Fatigue Syndrome, A Natural Healing Guide*. New York: Sterling Publishing Co., Inc., 1988.

PART IV

1. Woodman, Marion. *Addiction To Perfection*. Canada: Inner City Books, 1982. p. 13, 15.

- Perera, Sylvia Brinton. *Descent to the Goddess A Way of Initiation for Women*. Canada: Inner City Books, 1981.

SEVEN STATES of DEATH

Surrendering and Closing Down to the Outside World
1. St. John of the Cross. *Dark Night of the Soul*. New York: Doubleday, 1990. p. 66.

Surrendering the Physical Body
1. Steinem, Gloria. "Gross National Self Esteem." *Ms* (Vol. II, Number 3). p.26.

- Steinem, Gloria. *Revolution From Within, A Book of Self Esteem*. Boston: Little, Brown and Company, 1992.

Surrendering to Nothingness
1. Satprem. *By The Body Of The Earth*. New York: Harper & Row, 1978. p. 166.

2. Burton, Sandra. "Condolences, It's a Girl." *Time, Women: The Road Ahead* (Special Issue Fall 1990). p. 36.

Surrendering to the Witch Mother
1. Miller, Jean Baker. *Toward a New Psychology of Women*. Boston: Beacon Press, 1986. p. 4.

- Chernin, Kim. *Reinventing Eve, Modern Woman in Search of Herself.* New York: Times Books, 1987.

- Mason, Marilyn. *Making Our Lives Our Own.* San Francisco: Harpers, 1991.

Surrendering to the Shadow Father

1. Woodman, Marion. *Addiction To Perfection.* Canada: Inner City Books, 1982. p. 57.

2. Schafe, Ann Wilson. *Women's Reality, An Emerging Female System In A White Male Society.* New York: Harper & Row, 1985. p. 5.

3. Woodman, Marion. *Pregnant Virgin.* Canada: Inner City Books, 1985. p. 35.

4. Schafe, Ann Wilson. *Women's Reality, An Emerging Female System In A White Male Society.* New York: Harper & Row, 1985. p. 40.

5. Schafe. Ibid. p. 40.

6. Schafe. Ibid. p. 24.

7. Levine, Steven. "Conscious dying." *Utne Reader* (Sept./ Oct. 1991). p. 66.

- *Time, Women: The Road Ahead* (Fall 1990).

- Gilbert, Holle;, Laatz, Joan. "The rapists among us." *The Oregonian.* August, 8, 1991.

- "Why doesn't the U.S. have a Family Policy?" *Utne Reader* (Sept./Oct. 1991).

THE AWAKENING: THE SEVEN STATES of REBIRTH

The Decision to Live
1. Levine, Steven. "Conscious dying." Utne *Reader* (Sept./ Oct. 1991). p. 66.

2. Griffin, Susan. "Canaries in the Mine." *The Inquiring Mind* (May 1991). p. 4.

3. *A Course of Miracles*. Foundation of Inner Peace. 1977. p. 142.

4. Woodman, Marion. *The Pregnant Virgin*. Canada: Inner City Books, 1985. p. 47.

5. *A Course of Miracles*. Foundation of Inner Peace. 1977. p. 418.

6. *A Course of Miracles*. Ibid. p. 418.

7. Woodman, Marion. *The Pregnant Virgin* Canada: Inner City Books, 1985. p. 33.

• Chernin, Kim. *Reinventing Eve, Modern Woman in Search of Herself.* New York: Times Books, 1987.

Healing the Feminine Roots
1. Chernin, Kim. *Reinventing Eve, Modern Woman in Search of Herself.* New York: Times Books, 1987. p. xvi.

2. Eisler, Riane. *The Chalice & The Blade*. San Francisco: Harper & Row, 1987. p. xvii.

3. Gimbutas, Marija. "The First Wave of Eurasian Steppe

Pastoralists into Copper Age Europe," *The Journal of Indo-European Studies* (Winter 1977), p. 281.

4. Gimbutas, Marija. "Goddesses and Gods of Old Europe, 7000-3500 B.C. (*Berkeley and Los Angeles: University of California Press,* 1982), pp. 37-38.

5. Cameron, Ann. *Daughters of Copper Woman.* Canada: Press Gang Publisher, 1981. p. 60.

6. Cameron, Ann. Ibid. p. 102.

7. Cameron, Ann. Ibid. p. 102.

8. Cameron, Ann. Ibid. P. 61.

9. Cameron, Ann. Ibid. p. 62.

New Beginnings

1. Chernin, Kim. *Reinventing Eve, Modern Woman in Search of Herself.* New York: Times Books, 1987. p.xvii.

• Chopin, Kate. *The Awakening.* New York: Bantam Books, 1988.

• Pearson, Carol. *The Hero Within.* San Francisco: Harper & Row, 1986.

• Woolger, Jennifer; Woolger, Roger. *The Goddess Within., A Guide to The Eternal Myths That Shape Women's Lives.* New York: Fawcett Columbine, 1989.

The Emerging Woman

1. Woodman, Marion. *The Ravaged Bridegroom, Masculinity in Women.* Canada: Inner City Books, 1990. p. 18.

2. Milton, John. *The Student's Milton.* Rev. ed. Ed: Frank Allen Patterson. New York: Apple-Century-Crofts, Inc., 1933. Paradise Lost, line 299.

3. Woodman, Marion. "Feminine and the Wisdom of the Body." *Magical Blend* (January, 1992). p. 30.

4. Heilbrun, Carolyn G. *Writing A Woman's Life.* New York: Ballantine Books, 1988. p. 84.

5. Woodman, Marion. "Feminine and the Wisdom of the Body." *Magical Blend* (January, 1992). p. 30.

CONCLUSION

1. Starhawk. *Truth or Dare, Encounters With Power, Authority, And Mystery.* San Francisco: Harpers, 1987. p. 294.

2. Cooper, J.C. *An Illustrated Encyclopaedia Of Traditional Symbols.* London: Thames and Hudson, 1978. p. 156.

3. The Pantheon Fairy Tall & Folklore Library. *The Complete Grimm's Fairy Tales.* New York: Random House, 1972. p. 254.

BIBLIOGRAPHY

A Course in Miracles. Foundation of Inner Peace. 1977.

AMA. *The American Medical Association Encyclopedia of Medicine.* New York: Random House, 1989.

Boly, Williams. "Raggedy Ann Town." *Hippocrates* (July/ August 1987).

Burton, Sandra. "Condolences, It's a Girl." *Time, Women: The Road Ahead* (Special Issue Fall 1990).

Calhoun, Marcy. *Are You Really Too Sensitive? How to Develop & Understand Your Sensitivity as the Strength it is.* Nevada City, CA: Blue Dolphin Press, 1987.

Cameron, Ann. *Daughters of Copper Woman.* Canada: Press Gang Publisher, 1981.

Chernin, Kim. *Reinventing Eve, Modern Woman in Search of Herself.* New York: Times Books, 1987.

Chopin, Kate. *The Awakening.* New York: Bantam Books, 1988.

Conant, Susan. *Living With Chronic Fatigue, New Strategies for Coping With And Conquering CFS.* Texas: Taylor Publishing Co.1990.

Cooper, J.C. *An Illustrated Encyclopaedia Of Traditional Symbols.* London: Thames and Hudson, 1978.

DeFreitas, Hilliard, Brendan. "Association Of An HTSV-II-Like Virus With CFIDS." *The CFIDS Chronicle (Spring, 1991).*

DeFreitas, Elaine; Hilliard, Brendan; Cheney, Paul; Bell, David. "Retroviral sequences related to human T-lymphotropic virus type II in patients with chronic fatigue immune dysfunction syndrome." Proc. Natl. Acad. Sci. USA (Vol. 88. April 1991).

Eisler, Riane. *The Chalice & The Blade*. San Francisco: Harper & Row, 1987.

Heilbrun, Carolyn G. *Writing A Woman's Life*. New York: Ballantine Books, 1988.

Fisher, Gregg, Straus, Stephen, Cheney, Paul, Oleske, James. Chronic *Fatigue Syndrome, A Victim's Guide To Understanding, Treating, & Coping With This Debilitating Illness*. New York:Time Warner Books, 1987.

Gimbutas, Marija. "The First Wave of Eurasian Steppe Pastoralists into Copper Age Europe." *The Journal of Indo-European Studies*. (Winter 1977).

Gimbutas, Marija. "Goddesses and Gods of Old Europe, 7000-3500 B.C." (*Berkeley and Los Angeles: University of California Press*, 1982).

Griffin, Susan. "Canaries in the Mine." *The Inquiring Mind*. (May 1991).

Hendler, Sheldon. The *Oxygen Breakthrough 30 Days to an Illness-Free Life*. New York: William Morrow & Co., 1989.

King, Sheila. *Reiki House*. August 1991.

Klimas, Nancy; Salvato, Fernando; Morgan, Robert; Fletcher, Mary Ann. "Immunologic Abnormalities in

Chronic Fatigue Syndrome." Journal *of Clinical Microbiology,* (June 1990).

Landay, Alan; Jessop, Carol; Lennette, Evelyne; Levy, Jay. "Chronic fatigue syndrome: clinical condition associated with immune activation." *Lancet* (Vol. 338. No. 8769. Saturday 21, Sept. 1991).

Levine, Steven. "Conscious dying." *Utne Reader* (Sept./Oct. 1991).

Leviton, Richard. "What Does Illness Mean?" *Yoga Journal* (November/December 1991).

Mason, Marilyn. *Making Our Lives Our Own.* San Francisco: Harper and Row, 1991.

Murdock, Maureen. *The Heroine's Journey.* Boston & Shaftesbury: Shambhala, 1990.

Miller, Jean Baker. *Toward a New Psychology of Women.* Boston: Beacon Press, 1986.

Milton, John. *The Student's Milton.* Rev. ed. Ed: Frank Allen Patterson. New York: Apple-Century-Crofts, Inc., 1933.

Ostrom, Neenyah. "What Really Killed Gilda Radner?" New York: *The New Magazine,* Inc. 1991.

Pearson, Carol. *The Hero Within.* San Francisco: Harper & Row, 1986.

Perera, Sylvia Brinton. *Descent to the Goddess A Way of Initiation for Women.* Canada: Inner City Books, 1981.

Poesnecker, G.E. *Adrenal Syndrome, The Disease No Doctor Wants To Treat*. PA: Humanitarian Publishing Company, 1983.

Progoff, Ira. *At a Journal Workshop The Basic Test And Guide For Using The Intensive Journal*. New York: Dialogue House Library, 1975.

Sams, Jamie and Carson, David. *Medicine Cards: The Discovery Of Power Through The Ways Of Animals*. New Mexico: Bear and Company, 1988.

Satprem. *By The Body Of The Earth*. New York: Harper & Row, 1978.

Schafe, Ann Wilson. *Women's Reality, An Emerging Female System In A White Male Society*. New York: Harper & Row, 1985.

Smith, Barbara Leigh. *Married Women And The Law*. Bodichon, 1894.

Solomon, Neil. *Sick & Tired of being Sick & Tired*. New York: Wynwood Press, 1989.

Starhawk. *Truth or Dare, Encounters With Power, Authority, And Mystery*. San Francisco: Harper and Row, 1987.

Steinem, Gloria. "Gross National Self Esteem." *Ms* (Vol. II, Number 3).

Steinem, Gloria. *Revolution From Within, A Book of Self Esteem*. Boston: Little, Brown and Company, 1992.

St. John of the Cross. *Dark Night of the Soul.* New York: Doubleday, 1990.

Stoff, Jesse A., Pellegrino, Charles. *Chronic Fatigue Syndrome, The Hidden Epidemic.* New York: Random House, 1988.

The Pantheon Fairy Tall & Folklore Library. *The Complete Grimm's Fairy Tales.* New York: Random House, 1972.

Toor, Djohariah. *The Road By The River.* San Francisco: Harper & Row, 1987.

"Why doesn't the U.S. have a Family Policy?" *Utne Reader* (Sept./Oct. 1991).

Williams, Linda. "Stalking a Shadowy Assailant." *Time* (May 14, 1990).

Wilkinson, Steve. *Chronic Fatigue Syndrome, A Natural Healing Guide.* New York: Sterling Publishing Co., Inc., 1988.

Woolger, Jennifer, Woolger, Roger. *The Goddess Within., A Guide to The Eternal Myths That Shape Women's Lives.* New York: Fawcett Columbine, 1989.

Woodman, Marion. *Addiction To Perfection.* Canada: Inner City Books, 1982.

Woodman, Marion. *The Pregnant Virgin, A Process of Psychological Transformation.* Canada: Inner City Books, 1985.

Woodman, Marion. *The Ravaged Bridegroom, Masculinity in Women.* Canada: Inner City Books, 1990.

SWAN • RAVEN & COMPANY

The Swan and the Raven traditionally carry the
sacred message between the other world and our world.
Swan • Raven & Company publishes books whose
themes explore this sacred message.

To order additional copies of this book ($14.95 plus
$1.50 postage) or a catalogue, write or call:

Swan • Raven & Company
1427 N.W. 23rd Avenue, Suite 8
Portland, Oregon 97210

1-800 488-4849

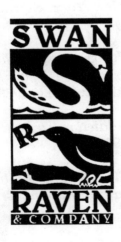